Autoimmune Protocol

Heal Your Body and Reverse Chronic Illness

(Eliminate Food Triggers on the Autoimmune Protocol)

Regina Carlson

Published By **Simon Dough**

Regina Carlson

Autoimmune Protocol: Heal Your Body and Reverse Chronic Illness (Eliminate Food Triggers on the Autoimmune Protocol)

ISBN   978-1-77485-783-0

Legal & Disclaimer

Table Of Contents

Chapter 1: Magic Of The Immune System

"When the impossible occurs, the lighthouse provides an indication of hope. If we are willing to accept hope it's all possible." -- Christopher Reeve

If you've been hearing the news about "Autoimmune Disease". ..." But what is that? This means that of 327 million Americans who are in those "lucky" 7.2 percent of people who have an immune system that attacks itself.

What is The Immune System?

The cause of sickness is the presence of toxins, bacteria or viruses that infiltrate the body, and also cells within the body that change. Without any defense against them and if we didn't, we'd be dead in a matter of minutes from even the most insignificant of substances. Our defense is composed of a complicated system of cells, organs, and tissues that work together to create our Immune System. The system initially defends against invaders like bacteria or viruses , and later attack if something should go through.

Your immune system consists of three types of immune system. They are intrinsic immunityof the body, acquired immunity and passive immunity.

These immunities form two immune systems that each have their own unique response. They are adaptive and innate immune response. Two different systems, but an immune system in one, communicate with one another in a variety of complex and vital ways. If they are not in balance it could have dire consequences.

The Innate System (Innate Immunity)

Your innate system generates your own immunity. That's your immunity the which you've always been blessed. It's the immune system's 2nd line of defense because it will immediately take on any thing it perceives to be an attack. This system reacts similarly to any threat, and is referred to as non-specific. It also responds to each disease in the exact manner. This is what makes the innate system sometimes referred to as non-adaptive. The elements of the natural system are:

* Stomach acid

* Phagocytic white blood cell

* Fever

* Enzymes found in your skin oils

* There are enzymes in your tears

* Inflammation

* Cough reflex

* Antimicrobial chemicals.

*Mucus (traps microscopic particles as well as bacteria)

A Adaptive Systems (Acquired Immunity)

The adaptive system generates the acquired immune system. It's your immune system's third line. Not only is it adaptable and adaptable, but it's also specific. This means it can tell the distinction between one pathogen and another and will respond in a particular way to each. Even though it could require an adaptive immune system short time to fight an infection the first time it comes across it, after fighting it for a while, it is able to recognize the weaknesses of the pathogen and will swiftly eliminate it the following time around if your immune system allows it to get back into the picture.

The primary parts that make up the immune system's adaptive systems are lymphocytes which , as we've learned previously, are a type composed of white blood cells. First, your B cells target an antigen (a pathogen fragment). Then, TH cells release the chemicals that activate to activate your B cell (immune Cell). This initiates

3

the chain reaction, which leads to the development of antibodies that kill the pathogen. Once the outbreak has ended the body converts only a tiny portion of activated TH and B cells in memory cells which protect you from the pathogen.

Passive Immunity

Passive immunity occurs by the use of antibodies that are produced outside your body. An example of this could include the immunity that a newborn gets from antibodies derived from the breastmilk. Another instance that passive immunity can be found is is acquired via an vaccination (antiserum injection) like the antitoxin tetanus. However in the case of passive immunity, although it offers immediate protection is not permanent. It requires repeated exposure. The benefits wear off.

What is the Immune System Work?

In the course of the day your system's immune response is in alert for something known as antigens. Antigens are foreign invaders that which the body identifies as dangerous. These could be bacteria, viruses or fungi. Drugs, chemicals, toxins and even eyelashes are recognized in the form of an antigen. They could be proteins (occasionally it's other things) on cells' surface. However, it's not the only thing the immune system must be looking for. Additionally, there are damaged cells known as free radicals within your bloodstream, which steal electrons from healthy cells, causing damage to them and potentially leading to diseases like cancer.

The body is awash with antigens, also known as HLA antigens which are believed to be present. They can be proteins which are a normal component in your cell. Your immune system recognizes these antigens as being normal and lets them to themselves. This is why we have to ask:

What is the best way to determine what to take on and what should be left alone?

Your body is incredible. The first step is to emit "danger" signals to signal their presence. They are referred to as"dangerous molecular patterns" (DAMPs). When your immune system is aware of the presence of a DAMP that comes in a variety of forms and forms, it can determine whether it wants to attack the cell and knows what it can do to target it. Since damaged cells could be the result of a range of conditions from sunburn to infections or cancer. Your body is in the middle of a task to do it.

Additionally contact with microbes that are infectious and pathogens set off a different sequence of signals. Infectious microbes are essentially viruses and bacteria. These signals are referred to as molecular patterns associated with pathogens (PAMPs). Each PAMP responds to in a different way.

The immune system also must deal with allergens such as pollen, fungi and food. The way that your body reacts to each one of these is dependent on the degree of an intruder it determines this particular allergen represents in your system. This is the reason why some people have no allergies in the first place.

Once your body is aware of the difference between a friend and something foreign, then what?

What is an immune reaction?

The immune response describes how your body reacts to antigens present in your system. The immune system in a healthy state is in full gear immediately fighting off the virus or fungi, bacteria, or virus the moment it is first attacked. If it's not triggered at the time it's needed or doesn't have enough resources to effectively eliminate the invader, you'll be faced with issues that include infection or illness. But, if the

6

immune system gets activated without reason or is unable to "shut off" when the threat has been eliminated, you can end up suffering from various issues, like an allergic reaction or autoimmune disease.

A major reason why an effective immune system functions so well is due to the fact that it's so broad. It's able to use nearly every aspect that is part of our body. Let's examine each component of your immune system, and how it reacts to the threat of invaders.

Skin

Your skin is the first protection. It's similar to the walls and motes all around your castle. Skin cells protect against viruses, bacteria, and other microbes through the release of antimicrobial proteins. These proteins attack microbes when they come into contact. The immune cells also grow in the various layers of the skin.

Bone Marrow

Each immune cell, even though they are different from one another, start their the process of life by forming stem cells in the bone marrow. They then travel to where they are. They then mature into the required immune cells. These mature cells, even though they come in the exact same place can then perform the function of immune for that area of the body.

The myeloid progenitor cell transforms into the innate immune cell that are cells that fight infections. These adaptive immune cells (B cells and T cells) that fight against specific bacteria and viruses develop in the lymphoid stem cells. Natural killer cells (NK cells) also develop from the lymphoid progenitor cell. NK cells are responsible for the functions of both innate and adaptive immune cells.

Bloodstream

The immune cells continuously monitor the bloodstream, and are ready to strike at the earliest sign of trouble. The immune cells found in your bloodstream are referred to as white blood cells or leukocytes. Doctors can determine whether your immune system has been stimulated by an infection caused by bacteria by checking neutrophils, which is one type of leukocyte.

There are two families of leukocytes--phagocytes and lymphocytes. Phagocytes fight off pathogens and kill what they can. Lymphocytes copy pathogen-related information inside the cell, so that it is remembered, and later removes the pathogen completely.

The two families consist of five different types of leukocytes and each performs their own immune system task.

* The one that was mentioned earlier, neutrophils are among the first immune defenses on the scene when confronted with an infection caused by microbial.

* Monocytes are among the first to respond to a bacteria-related infection. They are slower to respond and last for longer more so than neutrophils. They're also the initial response to an infection pathogen.

* Eosinophils are immune cells that fight multicellular parasites.

Basophils are the primary reaction to inflammation. They release chemicals like Histamine and heparin upon activation.

* Lymphocytes comprise B lymphocytes (B cells) and T lymphocytes (T cells). T cells and B cells cooperate to trigger the chain reaction, which leads to the creation of antibodies when they encounter bacteria and viruses. Cytotoxic T cells and NK cells work together to eliminate the virus-infected cells.

Antibodies

The antibodies produced by the Lymphocytes will then recognize damaged or infected cells and tagging them to be eliminated. However, it's not able to perform the destruction. This is the responsibility of NK cells.

Antibodies can also neutralize the effects of toxins (whether they're biological or pathological) and also activate the complement system that is a collection of proteins that aid in eliminating bacteria, viruses, or affected cells.

Complement

It is comprised up of more than thirty distinct proteins, which also work together to fight off antigens, specifically bacteria that cause infection. The liver is the organ responsible for the production of most of the components of the complement system. These proteins move through the body via extracellular blood and fluids, until they are required.

And only then the immune system sends two signals. One signal is generated by the molecules that are embedded within the microorganism. Another signal is activated by antibodies that are attached to the surface of the microorganism. If one complement is activated and activates the next two complements that follow. In this manner they generate two pathways, each of which leads towards an identical pivotal protein. If the pathways connect and the pivotal protein is activated, triggering an enraged assault on microorganisms.

Lymphatic system

It plays a significant role within the immunity system. It is made up consisting of extracellular fluid, lymphoid organs along with lymphatic blood vessels. It is among the main routes of travel between tissue and bloodstream.

The lymphatic vessels run throughout the body and transport toxic substances out of the body. They also hold lymphatic fluid and immune cellsthat make the lymph organs their home base.

These immune cells are on on this highway to perform the role of a reconnaissance. Since the lymphatic system transports the waste products from other cells it scans it for DAMPs and PAMPs. If they find something and the immune response within the cell will be activated. It will then reproduce and the cells will be released in huge numbers to smash and kill.

There are a variety of lymph organs that are part of the lymphatic system. These include bones marrow, lymph nodes the spleen, and the thymus.

Lymph Nodes

Along the highway that connects lymphatic vessels and immune cells, are a number of tiny "pathogen traps." These are designed specifically for the purpose of capturing and eliminating pathogens , other invaders, or damaged cells that they pass through these "traps" are known as lymph nodes. The lymph nodes are beans-shaped clusters of immune cells filled with white blood cells, which is every "invader's" most terrifying nightmare.

Thymus

The immune cells within the thymus are known as T cells. The thymus is among the smaller organs located in the upper chest near your thyroid.

Spleen

While the spleen's function isn't directly connected to the lymphatic system directly, it performs the same function and is a part of it in the same. It's an integral part of our body's defenses since it filters blood and relays the information it gathers. The spleen is also brimming in immunity system cells which are prepared to attack and activate when a pathogen that is blood-borne is detected.

Mucosal Tissue

One of the easiest entry locations to any bacteria or virus is through mucosal surface, which includes the nostrils, lips, ears the genital region eyelids, anus, and genital area. Our immune system has it covered. Our digestive, respiratory, and reproductive tracts covered with mucosal tissues. This is the tissue that keeps the insides inside and the outsides out. But how do you stop bacteria and viruses from crossing the threshold? It's your mucosal tissues, which does not just provide the barrier, but it also has some cells on alert. The gut has different areas with access points where immune cells monitor the content of the digestive tract to determine indications of alarm.

Inflammation

If your tissues are damaged due to the effects of trauma such as heat, bacteria or toxins, or any other antigen, the inflammatory reaction is triggered. The body will release various kinds of chemical. Some of them include prostaglandins, histamine and bradykinin. If these chemicals enter your system, blood vessels start to leak fluid into tissues that are damaged. This leads to inflammation around your antigen which aids in keeping it from other tissues.

The chemicals released by the inflammatory process also attract phagocytes. They do not just eliminate germs, but "eat" dead or damaged cells too. This is referred to as phagocytosis.

What is an altered immune Response?

Your immune system could produce one of three reactions: an effective immune response, an ineffective immune response, or the overactive response to your immune system. When your system's immune response is in good health, protecting you well and defending you adequately, then you have an effective immune response.

In the event that your system of immunity allows you to contract illnesses, then it's not working. If it's not caused by an external cause, such as medication, an inadequate immune system is usually due to an immune deficiency disorder. The condition of an immune deficiency could occur as a primary condition, which means that you have it as a result of birth or it, that is, it's caused by another disease.

Additionally, there is an active immune system. Hypersensitivity or allergic reactions could cause that your system's immune response to become hyperactive. This can lead to an autoimmune condition to develop. This is the point at which your immune system begins to attack the body. In both cases, an overactive and inefficient immune system has altered response.

How Come Your Immune System Start Attacking Your Body?

It wasn't until the start into the century of the twentieth century when Paul Ehrlich proposed that autoimmune tissue attacks could be possible. He was not convinced that the autoimmune reaction could develop into a pathological condition. In the 1950s, we finally were able to gain a better understanding of autoantibodies and autoimmune diseases in the way they are now.

We've come a long ways yet doctors do not have a solution to that question. They have observed that certain autoimmune disorders are more common in certain groups of people.

* A 2014 study published on sciencedirect.com found that two women have an autoimmune condition for each male.

* Autoimmune diseases generally kick off between the ages of 15 to the age of 44.

They tend to prefer one group of ethnicity over the other. For instance, Lupus tends to be more common in Hispanic as well as African Americans than Caucasians.

Certain autoimmune disorders tend to develop due to genetic. If for instance, one family member suffers from MS or lupus or multiple sclerosis, the other family members could develop an autoimmune condition also. This may not be the identical.

* Researchers suggest that you may be more likely to develop an auto-immune condition when exposed to certain chemicals, solvents or environmental elements.

* A study conducted during 2015, by Lisa A. Reynolds, Leah T. Stiemsma, B. Brett Finlay, and Stuart E. Turvey theorizes that the absence or exposure to germs could result in an overreactive response in the body to non-harmful antigens.

* A diet rich in fat and sugar and comprised of a great deal of processed food is believed to trigger inflammation. This causes an autoimmune reaction and increases the chance to develop an autoimmune condition. Therefore, the subject matter is the subject of the book.

A strong immune system is crucial for an overall healthy body. If the immune system isn't in balance, it not just does not have the ability to protect itself from antigens and viruses, but it may also begin self-attack, leading to an autoimmune condition that can be devastating to put it in a word. When this happens the immune system is more sensitive to everything around us. Simple things like vigorous exercise, pressure of personal issues travel, changing your food habits can impact the overall condition of your health. Additionally, prolonged exposure to even mild inflammation could increase your risk of developing additional diseases like cancer and cardiovascular disease.

Chapter 2: The Faces Of Autoimmune Disease

"And when the storm has passed you'll forget the way you got through, or how you were able to get through it. It's impossible to know for certain that the storm has ended. One thing is for certain. After you've emerged from the storm, you'll never become the exact person as when you was walking in. This storm is all about."

-- Haruki Murakami

Nowadays, it seems like that you can't turn on TV or check out social media without being informed about autoimmune disorders. I'm not sure how many of people I know are diagnosed one type of autoimmune disorder over the past decade. From rheumatoid to MS up to Graves" disease. Autoimmune conditions are everywhere. What does an individual mean by an autoimmune disorder? What is the cause? How do they get recognized and dealt with in the standard of medical practice? In this section, we're going to take a deep review of the much discussed but not always recognized autoimmune disease.

What is An Autoimmune Disease?

Have you been to the supermarket and noticed an acquaintance you haven't seen for a while? You walk up to the person and say "hi" and then touch them on the shoulder and then when they turn around you realize you've never seen this person before in person. They're a total stranger. You are in a state of anxiety when you are trying to think of something to say. Then the awkward explanations start.

Autoimmune disorders are similar to this illustration. To defend itself against viruses and bacteria our bodies have created an incredible and intricate security systems the immune system. The powerful security guards. This system is comprised of white blood cells. They guard the roads of the body , which is known as"the system of vascularization. The the vascular system is comprised of arteries and veins that transport circulation of blood away from the heart through the body, and returning to it. They are in constant patrol of the vascular system looking for invading organisms like germs and viruses. When they discover those "bad" cells in the vascular system, they begin to begin attacking. But, if someone suffers from an autoimmune disorder and these white blood cells misinterpret our cells as a harmful invading cell. Therefore, the white blood cells infiltrate the cells to attack the. The white cells could make a mistake with any of our types of organs, cells, or systems. After your white cells have recognized them as potentially dangersome, they will continue to attack these cells.

Close-up of Neutrophil Antibody (white blood cells)

If this occurs then you are suffering from an autoimmune condition. There are over eighty identified autoimmune disorders which affect more than 23 million Americans who suffer from them. About 80% of those who are diagnosed are females. Each autoimmune condition is a distinct system, body organ, or even cell white cells mistake for an intruder. For instance, in my case, which is, Psoriatic Arthritis, my body is attacking both my joint cells and skin.

However, why are autoimmune disorders more common for women? Do women have weaker bodies and are more susceptible to diseases?

In reality, the reverse is the truth. Women are blessed with a double X the chromosome. The X chromosome contains more than 1000 varieties of genes on it. While the Y chromosome contains just 100 genes. That means that if there's an indefective gene located on their X chromosomes the female's redundant gene located on the opposite X chromosome will be inserted to replace the gene in question. This reduces the risk of females being susceptible to X-linked disease, hereditary or infectious and makes them significantly live longer and longer lives than males. However, in the event of autoimmune

20

diseases, it is the XX chromosomes may be the problem.

This chromosome, known as the Xchromosome the place where you will find the genes that make up an immune system. What is the reason women are afflicted with problems with autoimmune diseases? Doesn't having an increased immune system beneficial? It's not. The X chromosome is actually the only chromosome not doubled by both males and women. To keep women's bodies from being a double-expressed version of genes on the X chromosome, the body's natural process stops (inactivates) duplicate genes that reside located on the chromosome. The body's smart system performs this activation in a sequence (usually 50/50 for each the X the chromosome). But there are times when it isn't able to stop an unrelated gene. It could also activate gene that is redundant in a strange manner (60/40 and 80/20). When the body activates genes in a bizarre manner, it's called "skewed gene activation". Women's biology is a hindrance in the case of the autoimmune diseases. Although doctors and researchers aren't certain why hormones produced by females tend to cause autoimmune disease in a certain way. It's normal to see the first signs of symptoms of autoimmune disease to manifest during puberty.

In my experience, the first time my hands frozen, and I was unable to use my fingers, was when I was 17 years old in my freshman year of college. I'd had a few eruptions in the form of "rashes" across my face throughout the course of my life which were thought to be due to dry skin. However, it wasn't until later I discovered that these occasional "rashes" were actually psoriasis, more than just dry skin. My fingers would freeze and I knew precisely what was going on. My grandmother had been watching me struggle and ultimately die from complications of the same illness. Instead of seeking help I chose to avoid any symptoms, and pretend that I had no problems. If I had visited a doctor at that time I might be able to prevent the degeneration of my body that would occur 13 years after. The earlier you tackle these autoimmune disorders, the better. In many cases, doctors can reduce or stop the progression of these diseases. This is vital since autoimmune diseases are degenerative.

There are some signs you should be looking for when you suspect you are suffering from an autoimmune condition. These signs include:

* Joint swelling

* Joint pain

* Abdominal Pain

* Chronic Diarrhea or constipation

* Swollen Glands

* Other chronic digestive problems

* Chronic Fevers

Trouble swallowing food or drinks

Unexplained Weight Loss or weight gain

* Skin Rashes and Other Skin Problems

* Chronic Fatigue or Exhaustion

If you are experiencing these symptoms, you should talk to your physician about them.

Furthermore, I would not suggest beginning AIP as a substitute for obtaining medical diagnosis. When I began this program I was in the care of a rheumatologist (I am still). He monitored my blood work for signs of malnutrition , and for indications that I was getting better. As I got better I began to improve, he gradually removed me from the medicines I no longer required. AIP is best used in conjunction with medical care, not to be used as an alternative to it.

Diagnose, Cause and Treatment

Many complain that it's difficult to receive an autoimmune disease diagnosis. This is an issue due to a variety of reasons. The diagnosis of an autoimmune condition isn't a straight and dry procedure. There isn't any specific blood test can tell you conclusively that you do not have any of these conditions. It's more of a process of searching for markers in the blood, observing symptoms and taking tissue samples in some instances. It is also a complex process due to the fact that many symptoms could be caused by other diseases and viruses. It can take time and patience to get the right diagnosis. I have found that having the correct doctor crucial. My rheumatologist was able diagnose me while my other doctors were not able to diagnose me.

Doctors and researchers don't understand the causes of autoimmune disorders. However. There is a checklist of factors that they believe are significant factors that contribute to the commonality between patients. The items include:

* Genetics

* Lifestyle

* Environmental Factors

* Stress

* Weight

* Diet

* Smoking

Autoimmune illnesses can differ drastically in the extent to which they impact those who suffer from them. Some people's lives are quite unaffected, while another person can be extremely affected. In many instances the severity of disease is related to the way of life and environmental factors. Being overweight and smoking cigarettes are known to make illnesses more serious. In addition anyone with a high-risk genetic link appears to have drew the wrong one when it comes to how severe the illness.

How can Autoimmune Diseases be treated?

Traditionally, autoimmune disorders can be treated using one or various methods. Doctors prescribing corticosteroids (steroids) and immunosuppressants and non-steroidal anti-inflammatory medications. There are a variety of drugs within every class of medicines. The type of medication a doctor prescribes will be based on the severity of your illness and the severity of your condition and how well your body's tolerance is to.

Corticosteroids

Corticosteroids (aka steroids) are synthetic medicines that mimic the hormone cortisol which your body produces. They're used to lessen swelling (this can be described as the body's method that is used to attack harmful or foreign cells within your body) and also to reduce the activities in the system of immune defense. By slamming down an immune system that is weakened by those suffering from an autoimmune condition, it is expected to lessen the symptoms of the illness. But, it results in an immune system that is compromised. The most commonly prescribed corticosteroids include prednisone and cortisone.

Immunosuppressants

Immunosuppressants are used for exactly what they sound, namely to suppress the immunity system. These medications are used for range of reasons such as autoimmune diseases as well as anti-rejection drugs to treat organ transplants. There are a variety that are immunosuppressants (including corticosteroids). What you're prescribed will depend on your illness and body's tolerance. Some types of immunosuppressants include Corticosteroids

* prednisone

* prednisolone

Janus kinase inhibitors

* tofacitinib

Calcineurin inhibitors

* Cyclosporine

MTOR inhibitors

* sirolimus

* methotrexate

IMDH inhibitors

* leflunomide

Biologics

* adalimumab

* certolizumab

* etanercept

* infliximab

* rituximab

Monoclonal antibodies

* basiliximab

This is not all-inclusive list of drugs available. It is more of an summary. Most often, doctors prescribe lifestyle changes and diet modifications too.

Different types of autoimmune diseases

Here, I'll give a brief overview of the most commonly reported immune-mediated diseases as well as a brief description of each. It isn't an attempt to diagnose a illness, since that should be performed by a licensed physician. It is just information that may be useful in identifying the possibility of a condition and in encouraging you to consult with your physician.

Celiac disease

Celiac Disease is an autoimmune illness that causes the sufferer to be unable to consume gluten. When you consume gluten your body will respond by triggering an autoimmune reaction which results in damage to the small intestinal tract. Gluten is a protein that can be found in grains. It is also present in household and medical products such as Chapstick as well as on the stamps made from glue.

Crohn's disease

It is an auto-immune condition with a bowel-related effect. It is a cause of irritation of the intestinal lining and wall of the digestive tract. It can be a painful condition, but it isn't typically life-threatening.

Endometriosis

Endometriosis is an auto-immune disease in the uterus. The uterine lining tissue to develop throughout the reproductive system, the uterus as well as other organs. It can result in severe pain, infertilityand excessive menstrual flow and miscarriages.

Eosinophilic Esophagitis (EoE)

Eosinophilic Esophagitis is an auto-immune condition that is triggered by food allergies. It is a cause of an inflammation in the stomach, as well as the growth of eosinophilic tissues. Eosinophilic cells comprise a form made of white blood cells that are specifically adapted to the stomach. If these cells accumulate excessively, they cause swelling, which can lead to further autoimmune reactions.

Fibromyalgia

Fibromyalgia can cause widespread discomfort, tenderness as well as insomnia and fatigue. It isn't classified as an autoimmune disorder, but it is co-morbid with a variety of immune-mediated illnesses. Fibromyalgia can cause depression or worsen it.

Graves" disease

Graves" disease is an autoimmune disorder which affects thyroid function. It causes the thyroid gland to produce excessive amounts of the hormone. . It is a cause of inability to handle the heat, stress as well as weight gain. Women suffer more frequently than males.

Juvenile diabetes (Type 1 diabetes)

Juvenile Diabetes (Type 1 , diabetes) is an auto-immune disorder which causes pancreas not to make enough insulin. It is the hormone which assists in the transfer of glucose into the cells. In the absence of insulin, glucose can accumulate in the body and could lead to the onset of coma or even death.

Lupus

Lupus is an autoimmune disorder that causes inflammation in many different organs in the body. There are three main forms of lupus: Systemic Lupus Erythematosus (SLE), Discoid lupus and Drug-induced lupus.

Lyme disease

It is an auto-immune disease that is caused through the bites of tick that is transmitted by deer.

MS (MS)

Multiple Sclerosis (MS) can be described as an autoimmune disorder that affects the brain as well as the spinal cord. The autoimmune reaction occurs when the body fights the myelin sheathing on the nerves, thereby slowing the transmission of brain signals to other areas of the body.

PANDAS (Pediatric Autoimmune Neuropsychiatric Disorders Related to Streptococcus).

PANDAS is an auto-immune disorder that affects teenagers and children following the onset of the strep throat virus or scarlet fever. The autoimmune reaction is psychosis that causes OCD and Tourette's style behavior, as well as aggression.

Psoriasis

Psoriasis can be described as an autoimmune disorder that affects the face. The autoimmune response can cause the appearance of red patches due to the excessive production of cellulite in skin.

Psoriatic Arthritis.

Psoriatic arthritis can be described as an autoimmune illness in which the body's autoimmune reaction to psoriasis causes joint pain, joint inflammation and mobility issues.

Rheumatoid arthritis (RA)

Rheumatoid arthritis (RA) is an autoimmune condition that can cause swelling, pain and mobility issues in joints.

Type 1 diabetes

It is an immune disorder that causes the pancreas not make enough insulin. The hormone insulin is one which assists in transferring insulin into blood cells. If insulin is not present, sugar can accumulate in the body and may cause an illness or even death.

Chapter 3: The Autoimmune System Diet

"The truth is that we're all slightly broken. We need to learn to accept our broken pieces Be kind and compassionate with others, as well as ourselves." Karen Salmansohn

T

There is no universal "autoimmune food regimen," per se. This is the reason this book is called "Autoimmune Protocol." The Autoimmune Protocol looks different for every person. I'll explain why in a minute.

There has been research, however showing that certain foods can benefit people suffering from an autoimmune disorder that includes Eosinophilic Esophagitis or Crohn's disease or Lupus and other food items could be harmful. I'm using "may" as well as "can" due to the fact that it is true that there are some items that must be altered in accordance with your body's requirements.

A registered dietician with a clinical background located in Boston in the Frances Stern Nutrition Center, Alicia Romano, RD, stated regarding the Autoimmune Protocol, "There will be generalizations that will necessitate individualization."

There are many popular autoimmune diets available including one called the Autoimmune Protocol Diet (AIP) being the most well-known. The AIP is often referred to as"the Paleo Autoimmune Protocol Diet. In this regard that we'll begin this chapter by taking a closer look on what is known as the Paleo Diet.

What is Paleo?

What were the diets of our ancestors during the Paleolithic period, which began around 10000 years ago? The way they ate would provide us the same advantages they experienced: less heart disease, obesity, diabetes. Why? This wasn't an issue until agriculture was introduced around 10,000 years ago. At this the body's genes were unbalanced to its diet. This genetic mismatch is a reason for many of the health conditions that are a result of lifestyle.

Our ancestral diet was comprised of vegetables, fish and meats that were lean as well as seeds, fruits and nuts. They ate only what they could gather from nature by hunting and gathering. Paleo simply means living and eating in the same well-balanced way as our ancestors lived in the Paleolithic time period. It's about living and eating wholeheartedly, which has been shown to bring about significant improvements in health as well as maintaining a healthy weight.

It is also known as the Paleo diet may also be referred to by the Stone Age diet, Paleolithic diet, caveman diet or hunter-gatherer's diet.

What are the recommended diets?

The recommendations for diets differ according to the commercial Paleo diet to the next. But all of them follow the same basic guidelines.

What can You Consume on Paleo?

This diet follows guidelines. It can be adapted to your requirements. This is due to the fact that food choices during the Paleolithic time period was different based on the area. They ate what they could find at the time and in the amounts needed to flourish in the climate of that specific area. Certain people ate high-carb, plant-based diets, while others ate mostly animal-based foods as well as other foods that were low in carbs. However, their diets included a lot of wild-caught fish and seafood, fruits, vegetables and seeds as well as healthy fats and oils as well as eggs (you must consume free-range eggs) and fruits, herbs and vegetables, lean meat as well as nuts and spices. Since this is not an LCHF diet it is permitted to consume tubers, too that includes potatoes, yams, turnips or sweet potatoes. Whatever you choose to do in all your choices of food, you should make sure you choose the most minimally processed options that are with your spending budget.

Every now and then it is okay to indulge in a tiny amount of wine or dark chocolate is good. Red wine is loaded with antioxidants. If you're a lover of dark chocolate, which has numerous health benefits, it is important to select one with 70% cocoa in it percent or more.

What is the best food you can eat on Paleo?

It is essential to avoid everything Paleolithic human race didn't have readily available to them. This includes today's processed food items (including those labeled "low fat" or "diet") and beverages with artificial sweetness and trans-fats as well as margarine. However, it could also include thingslike:

*High-Fructose Corn Syrup

* Sugar

* Fruit Juices

* The majority of dairy-based product (some Paleo versions include full-fat dairy)

*Grains (including pasta and bread), spelt, barley and Rye)

* Legumes

* Salt

* A few oil-based vegetable products (sunflower oil as well as soybean oil, grapeseed oil oil cottonseed oil and safflower oil along with other oils)

* Certain variations of Paleo don't permit potatoes.

An easy guideline here is that if the food appears like it was made in a factory, it's probably not Paleo. Eat your food fresh.

A typical day's menu

Breakfast

2 Eggs 2 Eggs, 1 1/2 Cup of Tomatoes, 1/2 Green Peppers along with half Cup of Broccoli Fried in Coconut Oil

1. Cup Cantaloupe (cubed)

Snack

Carrot Sticks

Lunch

The Chicken Salad drizzled in Olive Oil

One Handful Of Nuts

Snack

1 Orange

Dinner

Ground Beef Stir-fry and vegetables

1 Handful Berries

Snack

- Celery Sticks

Drink plenty of fluids and engage in lots of physical activity.

Modified Paleo Diets

As I've stated that there are many variations that follow the Paleo diet available. In addition many people are now looking towards Paleo as a model to begin with. Therefore, they develop "Modified Paleo-based diets." They could comprise gluten-free grains (rice for instance) as well as other foods which are deemed healthy by science.

What is The Autoimmune Protocol Diet?

It is a form of diet that AIP is a variant that follows the Paleo diet at its extreme, which is mainly restricted to nutrient-rich foods like meats and vegetables with a focus on meats that contain omega-3 fats. It's designed to ease the symptoms that are associated with an autoimmune disease through healing the gut reduce inflammation. This is a new technique.

Researchers have discovered that some individuals might have tiny holes within their intestines that allow certain nutrients digested by the food to enter the body. This is referred to as "leaky stomach." The leaky gut can trigger the immune system to react, since it recognizes the foods in the form of an antigen. The AIP diet can help heal leaky gut.

AIP AIP can be described as an elimination-oriented diet that is designed to eliminate the cause of inflammation. The first step is to eliminate all foods that could cause inflammation. This will reset your immune system and puts it in Remission.

You adhere to the AIP diet for a few weeks, removing everything else. Then, you start adding other foods one at one at a time. The food additions are spread out by a few days up to the span of a week. In this way, if you have a reaction to a food that you are aware of the food that has caused it and you can keep it off of your diet.

There is no test that is reliable to identify the "best" food choices for every person. According the research of Zhaoping Li, MD, Ph.D., you must find it out on your own. Nobody is alike. The words of his father are "We must live and grow." But we know that certain foods that are not consumed.

Why are certain foods avoided?

We've been aware of the impact of our diet on our general health for a long time because it affects our energylevels, provides us with the nutrients we require to repair our cells and much more. However, it wasn't until fifty years ago when an connection between autoimmune diseases that cause inflammation along with diet was suggested. In recent years, it's becoming evident how much of a role our diet plays in the likelihood of developing of autoimmune diseases that cause inflammation.

With increasing numbers of people dining out and eating processed food items, the risk of autoimmune disorders is rising. This is due to diets that are low in omega-3 fatty acids and high in omega-6 fatty acids, which don't contain sufficient vegetables and fruits (and consequently, fiber) and include all grains, sugars, or processed carbs cause inflammation. Inflammation increases the chance of developing an autoimmune disease. If you already suffer from an autoimmune condition it can be a reason why they are more severe.

Sugar increases pain levels. It is a typical manifestation of an autoimmune condition. It appears to occur in conjunction with inflammation. Both of these are exacerbated by sugar intake. It's not just that cutting down on sugary drinks, desserts and drinks that contain sugar lessen the symptoms and symptoms, but eating AIP-approved food items, like blueberries, spinach, and blueberries could actually boost levels too!

Dairy and gluten can trigger symptoms to worsen. The food sensitivities as well as food allergy can trigger an immune reaction. A lot of people are unaware of food sensitivities or allergies. If they consume the foods they are allergic or sensitive to, and the body responds to it, it can lead further towards developing an autoimmune disorder. If they already suffer from one eating these foods can cause more symptoms. But, removing the most common allergens, such as gluten and dairy and substituting them with AIP permitted foods can facilitate healing.

What foods should be avoided?

Since it is a very small list, it's no surprise that the "Thou Shalt Not Touch" list is extremely lengthy.

We've covered a few of the food items that I have listed as items to avoid on people following the Paleo diet. But, there are quite some more to avoid:

* Legumes (peanuts, soy, beans, hummus, etc.)

* Gum

* Tomatoes

* Potatoes

* Eggplant

* Sugar

* Corn syrup with high-fructose content

* Alternative sweeteners

* Food additives

* Nuts and seeds

* Chocolate

*All Grains (such as wheat, oats, or rice)

Certain spices belong part of the family of seeds (for instance, cumin and coriander)

• Emulsifiers, Thickeners and Thickeners

* Foods packaged or processed

* Peppers

* Dairy items (This is raw milk products!)

* Coffee

* Eggs

* Canola Oil

* Vegetable Oil

* Alcohol

* Trans-fats

Researchers suggest that you stay clear of nonsteroidal anti-inflammatory medications (NSAIDs). They are a class of painkillers. They comprise Bufferin (aspirin), Advil (ibuprofen) and Aleve (naproxen sodium).

It is also recommended to stay clear of blue-green algae. Blue-green algae could cause an immune response. Therefore, it is recommended to avoid those suffering from an autoimmune illness.

What are the reasons certain foods are included?

There are a variety of foods that are on the AIP approved list. The list is there for reasons. They're not just a random suggestion. The basis is an idea of the Paleo food plan, they've been altered for a variety of health reasons.

1. A diet known as the Autoimmune Protocol Diet increases insulin sensitivity.

Researchers have discovered a connection between the autoimmune disorder insulin resistance. This not only increases the risk to develop an disease and aggravates symptoms too.

Insulin is among the most vital hormones found within your body. It is used by your body to regulate the amount of energy created through the consumption of carbs. If you consume a lot of carbs or eat a lot of sugar the body responds through the release of insulin huge quantities. In time your cells become adjusted to the insulin's effects and stop responding as they would.

If you consume the AIP diet, you can boost the sensitivity of your insulin! The food items that trigger this feat are the fiber found in fruits and vegetables, the healthy fats, as well as phytonutrients.

2. The AIP boosts the microbiome.

Research has shown that a weakened gut microbiome can cause inflammation and a weakened immune response. Because the trillions of microbes in your gut microbiome impact the capacity of your body to absorb nutrients and influence your immune system and because an imbalance can increase the likelihood for developing an auto-immune disease the enhancement of the microbiome of your body is essential.

When processed foods, sugar and grains create the perfect environment for bad bacteria to flourish The AIP eliminates bad bacteria. It boosts the microbiome within your gut by providing your good bacteria with the nutritional fiber they require.

3. AIP food items are loaded with nutrients needed to reduce inflammationand lower the chance of developing immune-related diseases, or improving present symptoms!

Researchers have discovered that a diet high in selenium, calcium vitamin A, D, and E and omega-3 fatty acids can help reduce inflammation. However zinc deficiency could increase your chances for developing an auto-immune disorder. People with autoimmune disorders are often lacking in (or at the very least, have low levels in) Iodine, copper selenium, potassium, zinc vitamin B, iron magnesium, chromium and.

The foods listed on the Autoimmune Protocol are rich macronutrients as well as micronutrients. It is essential to take both to reduce your chance for developing an autoimmune disorder and to alleviate any existing symptoms!

What foods should be included?

We've covered all the "Thou must not"s. Let's discuss the options available. The goal is to eliminate and replace. That means you're eliminating unhealthytrigger foods that cause inflammation in exchange for healthier whole food items. You ought to be eating plenty of meat and veggies, nightshade and other vegetables are not included Of course. Fruits are often included in small quantities.

Your list includes:

* Fish and seafood that are fatty

* Leafy green vegetables

* Meat

* Fruit (in tiny quantities)

* Herbs that are fresh (excluding seeds)

* Coconut milk

Extra virgin olive oil

* Avocado oil

* Coconut oil Extra Virgin

* Sweet potatoes

* Green tea

* Bone broth

* Maple syrup or honey (occasionally but only in tiny amounts)

* Dairy-free foods that are fermented (i.e. sauerkraut, nondairy Kefir, Kombucha, kimchi)

* Coconut

* The majority of Vinegars (must be free of sugar)

* Arrowroot starch

* Gelatin is made from grass-fed beef

Note: Fruits remain a subject of controversy. Some scientists will inform that you should cut out fruit completely, while others suggest that you should consume as much as 25g of fructose a day.

Conclusion

The Autoimmune Protocol Diet will reduce the body's inflammation which can reduce the chance that you will develop an autoimmune condition or ameliorate the symptoms of autoimmune disease when you already suffer from one. However, autoimmune disease management does not look the same way for everyone--particularly when it comes to managing it with AIP.

It is important to note that the Autoimmune Protocol Diet is not an all-inclusive diet. It is a custom-made diet to suit the individual's unique immune system.

The best method to keep track of what you've eaten , and when , so you can are aware of what your body reacts to and doesn't as you begin to incorporate things into your diet is keeping a food diary. It's easy to complete. Simply keep track of what you eat, and any reactions your body experiences. This will allow you pinpoint the triggers. Also, you'll be able to keep an accurate record of what you've tried to incorporate and what you've left out. A dietician may be able to assist you in this.

The process of understanding, preventing as well as treating an autoimmune disorder can be a challenge. I'm aware of how difficult it is to understand how the Autoimmune Protocol Diet looks. It looks restrictive and is. But you can do it. The reward is worth the effort. You're worth it.

Your family is dependent on to be healthy and worth it.

The AIP is known to reduce the chance for developing an immune disorder and ease the symptoms if you suffer from it. The AIP diet, along with lifestyle adjustments, like getting the proper amount of sleep, drinking plenty of water, and taking in sufficient vitamin D, is the most important measure to manage an autoimmune disorder. The benefits are far greater than the challenges of adhering to the AIP.

Chapter 4: Autoimmune Protocol Recipe

I'll admit it, for me, trying to cook on AIP AIP diet was a little difficult initially. The ingredients and techniques weren't the same as what I was doing in my cooking routine. But, as I delved involved in making food to prepare for AIP further, the methods came to be second nature to me. I don't cook nearly as often as I used to , but the times I cook I am truly enjoying cooking. Here are a few of my favorite recipes which you can test to see if you like them.

BREAKFAST RECIPES

Blueberry Coconut Smoothie recipe

by Louise Hendon

INGREDIENTS:

1 individual size container made of Coconut Milk Yogurt (blueberry or vanilla flavor)

2 Teaspoons of raw Honey

1/2 Cup Coconut Milk

1/2 - 3/4 Cups of fresh Blueberries

The Vanilla Extract is a Taste

A Handful of Ice

INSTRUCTIONS:

Step 1.

Put the coconut yogurt and blueberries, coconut milk, vanilla extract, and honey in the blender.

Step 2.

Mix well.

Banana Pancakes

Through: Paleo Flourish

INGREDIENTS:

1/2 Bananas,

1/4 Coconut Flour

1/8 Baking Soda

1 Tbs Coconut Oil

1 Tbs 1 Tbs. Honey or Maple Syrup

1 Tbs Gelatin

3TBs of water

INSTRUCTIONS:

Step 1.

Peel and put half of a banana that is ripe into the bowl.

Step 2.

The coconut flour should be added to mix bowl.

Step 3.

Incorporate baking soda along with coconut oil, baking soda, and honey or maple syrup.

Step 4:

Mix well to form a firm dough.

Step 5:

Create tiny ball (about about the same size as the size of a golf ball) made from dough. Form them into pancakes that are flat (about one-quarter inch). Set them on a parchment lined baking sheet. Place them in a 350 degree oven.

Step 6:

The baking time is 20 minutes. Take the oven out and allow to cool until be set. Serve with additional sweet maple syrup or honey.

https://healingautoimmune.com/easy-aip-recipes

https://paleoflourish.com/paleo-aip-banana-pancakes-recipe

AIP Flatbread Recipe

INGREDIENTS

1.25 Cups Coconut Flour

1 Cup Cassava Flour

2 teaspoons baking powder

1 Tablespoon Garlic Powder

1 Teaspoon of Mixed Dried Herbs

A generous pinch of salt

1 Tablespoon Nutritional yeast flakes

Half Cup Hot Boiling Water Boiling

3. Tablespoons Gelatin Powder

Three Tablespoons of Lukewarm Water

3 Tablespoons hot water

2 Tablespoons Olive Oil

Sea salt flakes to serve

INSTRUCTIONS

Preheat the oven to 350 F.

Step 1.

Blend the flours of coconut, sugar, cassava baking powder, garlic powder dried herbs, and salt in the bowl. Place the bowl on the table.

Step 2.

In a separate bowl dissolve the nutritional yeast pieces into warm water that is boiling. Set aside.

Step 3.

Sprinkle the gelatin powder on top of the cool water in an individual bowl. For for about 60 seconds, and then pour in the boiling water, and stir thoroughly to dissolve. Mix this gelatin solution that is dissolved in the nutritional yeast solution. Add olive oil. Whisk it well.

Step 4:

Mix the wet ingredients into the flour mixture, and mix with an wooden spoon. The mixture should be like an even dough. If it's dry and crumbly add some more water.

Step 5:

The dough should be divided into five equal-sized portions , then form them into balls. Place each ball on a baking sheet that is lined with parchment paper. Press into an oval shape that is about 1/2-inch thick.

Step 6:

In the oven, bake for 12 to 15 minutes, rotating the baking sheet half way through. Take it off and let it cool slightly. Add sea salt.

https://healingautoimmune.com/aip-flatbread-recipe

AIP Coconut Shrimp and Grits Recipe

INGREDIENTS

15 Button Mushrooms Diced

2. Cloves Garlic, Peeled and Minced

9oz Uncooked Shrimp, Peeled

Generous Squeeze Lemon Juice

1 Cup Coconut Cream

2/3 Cup unsweetened Desiccated Coconut

2 Tablespoons Flat-Leaf Parsley, Sliced (Optional) for Garnish

Crispy Bacon Bits (optional)

Salt to Taste

INSTRUCTIONS

Step 1.

The olive oil should be heated in an oil cooking pan. Add the garlic and mushrooms, and cook for 5 minutes.

Step 2.

Add the shrimp, and simmer until shrimp are pink. Incorporate the juice of the lemon and sprinkle salt. Set aside.

Step 3.

Make the coconut grits by heating the coconut desiccated in coconut cream.

Step 4:

Serve by placing the mushrooms and shrimp on the coconut "grits".

Garnish with bacon and parsley chunks (optional).

https://healingautoimmune.com/aip-coconut-shrimp-grits-recipe

Sweet Potato Breakfast Hash

INGREDIENTS

1 Sweet Potato 1 Sweet Potato, Shredded

1/2 Zucchini Shredded

1 Cup Meat Leftover, Shredded

1 Tablespoon fresh Thyme Leaf Finely chopped (Or Make use of 1 Teaspoon dried Thyme or other herbs of your choice)

1 Tablespoons Coconut Oil for cooking

Salt to Taste

INSTRUCTIONS

Step 1.

Coconut oil is heated on medium-high heat, and then add the sweet potato shredded as well as the zucchini that has been shredded. the meat left over.

Step 2.

Bake until sweet potato becomes tender (approx. 5 minutes).

Step 3.

Add the herbs to the mix and add salt according to your preference.

https://paleoflourish.com/sweet-potato-breakfast-hash-recipe-paleo-aip-gf

Raspberry Fillets of Breakfast Pastry

By Kelsey McReynolds

INGREDIENTS

Dough:

1 Cup Tapioca Flour

1 Cup Cassava Flour

1 Cup Coconut Sugar

3/4 Cup Hot Water

1/2 Cup Avocado Oil

Filling:

3 to 4 cups Raspberries (I used frozen)

3. Tablespoons Maple Syrup

The Juice from One Lemon

2-3 Scoops Vital Proteins Beef Gelatin

Glaze:

Coconut Butter, Melted

INSTRUCTIONS

Step 1.

In a medium-sized pot with a medium-low setting, mix the juice of a lemon, raspberries as well as maple syrup. Reduce the temperature to about 15 minutes, stirring frequently.

Step 2.

Add gelatin. Mix until there aren't additional chunks.

Once it has thickened up, take it off from the heat and allow it to cool prior to moving on.

Step 3.

Preheat oven at 350 degrees F.

Step 4:

In a bowl make a mix of coconut sugar, flours, avocado oil, hot water.

Step 5:

Knead dough until it is well-mixed.

Step 6:

With a rolling pin make a small amount of dough between two pieces of parchment. Make sure that it's about 1/2 inch thick.

Step 7:

Cute into a large rectangle, about 6x4 inches.

Step 8:

Scoop 1-2 teaspoons of raspberry mixture on one portion of dough. Be sure not to spread it over edge of dough. If you fill it too much, it won't be sealed properly.

Step 9:

Utilizing this parchment, guide one end of the dough until it meets the opposite side, and then enclosing it with the filling of raspberry. It should be now about 3x2.

Step 10.

Pin the edges or use an fork's tines press against the edges.

Step 11:

Place them carefully on a parchment-lined baking sheet. They are very delicate, therefore be extremely cautious.

Step 12:

Bake for approximately 15 minutes.

Step 13:

Serve your dish off with coconut butter, and serve!

https://autoimmunewellness.com/raspberry-filled-breakfast-pastry/

Paleo Pumpkin Donuts with Carob Frosting

by Michelle Hoover

INGREDIENTS

3/4 Cup Tigernut Flour

1/4 cup Coconut Flour

3. Tablespoon Tapioca Starch (Sub Arrowroot)

1/4 cup pumpkin puree

1/4 Cup Maple Syrup

1/4 Cup Coconut Milk

2. Tablespoon Coconut Oil

2 Teaspoon Cinnamon

1 Teaspoon Baking Powder

Gelatin Eggs for the Gelatin Egg

1 Tablespoon Gelatin

1/4 Cup Water

Optional Frosting: Optional Frosting

1/4 Cup Palm Shortening

2. Tablespoon Coconut Milk

2. Teaspoon Maple Syrup

1 Tablespoon Carob

Instructions

Step 1.

Preheat the oven until 350 F and then prepare the donut pan made of silicone.

Step 2.

Blend the Tigernut flour coconut flour, the coconut flour, and tapioca starch into one large bowl. Then, sift the ingredients

Step 3.

Add the pumpkin puree, maple syrup and coconut milk. Add cinnamon, coconut oil and baking powder. Stir until everything is well blended

Step 4:

To make the gelatin, eggs set a small pan on the stove , along with 1 cup of water. lightly sprinkle in 1 tablespoon gelatin. Mix until there is no lumps or clumps. Let the gelatin set for a couple of minutes.

Step 5:

Switch the stove to low to melt the gelatin. It will take about a minute. Don't let it get too hot.

Step 6:

Remove the mix from the heat and employ a whisk or blender to mix vigorously until it's smooth.

Step 7:

Incorporate the gelatin egg into the pumpkin mixture , and mix it all together right away.

Step 8:

Scoop the batter onto the baking pan. Then be sure to spread it evenly so that you don't risk breaking.

Step 9:

Bake for 35 to 40 minutes.

Step 10.

Take them out of the oven and let them cool for about 15 to 20 minutes inside the dish. Once they've cooled put an ice rack (or plates) on the top of the donut pan and turn it upside down to take the donuts off. Scooping them up with a spoon can smash them.

Step 11:

Let the donuts cool for an additional 10-15 hours on the rack for cooling.

Step 12:

For frosting that you can make mix the frosting components in a tiny bowl until they are well blended.

Step 13

Spread the frosting over donuts when they are cool to the point of contact.

Apple Cinnamon Granola

by Rebecca Boucher

Ingredients

2 Cups Toasted Coconut Flakes OR Tigernut Flakes

Half Cup of Apple Chips Crushed

1/3 Cup Raisins

2 Teaspoon Cinnamon

Pinch Salt with a Generous Pinch

1/4 Cup Coconut Oil, Melted or Avocado Oil

2. Tablespoon Maple Syrup

Half Tablespoon Arrowroot Powder

Instructions

Step 1.

Mix coconut, Tigernut flakes with apple chips as well as raisins, cinnamon as well as salt, in one large bowl. place aside.

Step 2.

A small bowl make a mixture of oil, maple syrup, and arrowroot until the arrowroot disintegrates.

Step 3.

Pour the oil mix over the dry ingredients, then combine until evenly.

Step 4:

Spread out on a parchment lined baking sheet.

Step 5:

Bake at 300 degrees for 30 minutes or until crisp and toasty.

The best AIP Waffles You've Ever Had!

by angelslice

Ingredients

2. Whole Plantain, Ripe

3/4 Cup Tigernut Flour

3/4 Cup Butternut Squash, Puree

1 Cup organic Coconut Oil It is melted

Half Teaspoon Baking Soda

12 Teaspoon Creme of Tartar

1 Tablespoon ground cinnamon

1 Pinch Sea Salt

Instructions

Step 1.

Switch on the waffle iron

Step 2.

Peel and place chopped plantains in the processor. Pulse briefly.

Step 3.

Add the remaining ingredients and blend until thoroughly blended. This batter should be thick and bubbly.

Step 4:

Pour the batter onto the waffle iron using a large Tablespoon full. Cook for 6 minutes per time.

Apple Cinnamon Roll Porridge with Coconut Butter Drizzle

by: Caitlin Sherwood

Ingredients:

1/4 cup Coconut Flour

12 Cup Boiling Water

1/2 Teaspoon Cinnamon

1/8 Teaspoon Vanilla

1 Tablespoon Honey (Optional)

3/4 Cup Cinnamon Apples

Coconut Butter To Use

Raisins for sprinkling (Optional but it adds good texture)

Instructions

Step 1.

Blend the coconut flour, and cinnamon using an fork in a tiny bowl.

Step 2.

Pour about half the water and continue to stir. The rest of the water, in a small amount at each at a time until the porridge is at the consistency you prefer (it should look a bit similar to oatmeal). If the porridge becomes too thick after some time, you can add additional water.

Mix in vanilla and honey.

Step 3.

Sprinkle with raisins and cinnamon apples, and drizzle coconut butter.

The Cinnamon Apples are for:

1 Tablespoon Coconut Oil

1 Crisp Apple

1/4 Teaspoon Cinnamon

Instructions:

Step 1.

The coconut oil is heated in a pan.

Step 2.

While the apple is heating, cut and core your apple.

Step 3.

Place the apple slices in the cooking pan, in an uniform layer. Cook with a stirring every now and then for 7 to 10 minutes.

Step 4:

Once the apples are soft mix in the cinnamon. Mix thoroughly, till the cinnamon has been evenly spread. Remove the stove from the heat.

https://www.forageddish.com/blog/2014/9/17/apple-cinnamon-roll-porridge-with-coconut-butter-drizzle

LUNCH RECIPES

Bacon Ranch Chicken Poppers

By: Michelle Hoover

INGREDIENTS

1 Pound Ground Chicken (or Turkey) Ground chicken (Or Turkey)

2 Cups of Raw Shredded Carrots (Shredded in a Food Processor or bought pre-Shredded)

3 Slices of Bacon, Raw, Sugar-Free

2. Tablespoon Coconut Oil

2. Tablespoon Coconut Flour

2. Tablespoon Dried Parsley

2 Teaspoons Dried Chives

1 Tablespoon Garlic Powder

1. Teaspoon Dried Dill

2. Teaspoon Onion Powder

1. Teaspoon Sea Salt

INSTRUCTIONS

Step 1.

Preheat the oven until 400 F and then line an oven sheets with parchment.

Step 2.

Place the carrots that have been shredded in a food processor , along together with bacon. Blend until smooth. The bacon and carrots require to be carefully chopped. Take the bacon and carrots from the food processor , and then add to the mixing bowl.

Step 3.

Mix in the ground chicken that is raw (or turkey) along with the seasonings, coconut oil and flour. Mix thoroughly.

Step 4:

Make small poppers, then slightly flatten them (you'll get 25-30 poppers)

Step 5:

Bake for 30 to 35 hours, turning them half way through. Put them in the oven for 5 minutes, until crispness before serving if you want,

Serve warm and warm with a smooth ranch dressing, and then take your time!

71

https://unboundwellness.com/bacon-ranch-chicken-poppers/

Chicken Reshmi Kebabs

By: Bethany

INGREDIENTS

1. Small Red Onion

2 Cloves Garlic

A Good Sense of Cilantro Leaves

1/4 Cup Plantain Chips

1 Teaspoon Pink Salt

1/2 Teaspoon Turmeric

1/4 Teaspoon Mace

1. Teaspoon Ginger Powder

1 Pound of Ground Chicken (Or chicken breasts cut into cubes)

2. Tablespoons Coconut Cream

1 Tablespoon Coconut Oil

INSTRUCTIONS

Step 1.

Put the onion as well as garlic and cilantro in the food processor and process until the mixture is smooth and begins to develop.

Step 2.

Incorporate the chips of plantain, and process until the chips are finely chopped.

Step 3.

Add chicken, spices, as well as coconut cream. Process until the entire mixture is blended and chicken is perfectly ground.

Step 4:

Divide the chicken mixture into 8 pieces and wrap around the skewers.

Step 5:

Place in the refrigerator to chillor set in 20 minutes.

Step 6:

In a large skillet on medium temperature.

Step 7:

Cook the kebabs for 3-4 mins for each side (total 10 to 15 minutes time to cook). The chicken should be cooked to perfection and the outside to turn brown.

Step 8:

Take them off the skewers.

http://adventuresinpartaking.com/2019/05/chicken-reshmi-kebabs/

Hawaiian Teriyaki Chicken Burgers

By: MICHELLE

INGREDIENTS

To make the Teriyaki Sauce

1 Cup Coconut Aminos

2. Teaspoon Coconut Sugar

2. Tablespoon Pineapple Juice

1. Teaspoon Arrowroot Starch

1 Teaspoon Sea Salt

The Burgers

1 Pound Ground Chicken

1. Tablespoon Coconut Aminos

1. Tablespoon Coconut Flour

1 Tablespoon Avocado Oil

1/2 Teaspoon Cumin

1. Clove Garlic Minced

1. Teaspoon Sea Salt

4 to 5 Slices of Pineapple

Half Red Onion, Sliced

8-10 Butter Lettuce Leaves (Optional)

1 Tablespoon Cilantro Chopped

INSTRUCTIONS

Step 1.

Mix all of the elements (except Arrowroot) into a tiny pot and place it on the stove over moderate temperature.

Step 2.

Whisk the arrowroot mixture at a low temperature for 3-4 minutes until the sauce begins to thicken. Keep it in the fridge.

Step 3.

The grill or the skillet by using avocado oil. Turn the heat up to medium-high.

Step 4:

In a bowl, mix the chicken's carcass with coconut aminos and coconut flour avocado oil and cumin, garlic and salt.

Step 5:

Mix thoroughly until completely mixed.

Make 4-5 burgers, then put them on the grill or on the pan.

Step 6:

Cook for 4-5 minutes both sides before carefully flipping. Cook until the internal temperature reads at 165 F. Place aside.

Step 7:

Clean the pan, and then add oil. Add the pineapple slices , and grill for about a minute on each side. This will create grill marks.

Set 8:

Put aside then repeating the recipe with the onion and red for two minutes each. Put the onion on the side.

Step 9:

To build the burgers place each patty on top of a leaf of lettuce and add pineapple the red onion, sauce teriyaki and cilantro.

https://unboundwellness.com/hawaiian-teriyaki-chicken-burgers-paleo-whole30-aip/

Shrimp Chimichangas

by: Jacqueline Martin

Ingredients

Tortillas

2 Cups Cassava Flour

6. Tablespoon Extra Virgin Olive Oil Extra Virgin

1/2 Teaspoon Pink Himalayan Sea Salt

1 Cup Water

"Cheese" Sauce

1 Head Cauliflower Chop

1 Cup Chicken Bone Broth

1 Cup Coconut Milk

4. Tablespoon Nutritional Yeast

1 Teaspoon Onion Powder

Half Teaspoon Garlic Powder

1 Teaspoon Dried Basil

Half Teaspoon Dried Oregano

1/2 Teaspoon Pink Himalayan Sea Salt

Shrimp

2 Pounds Shrimp Raw Peeled

1 Medium Onion Diced

2. Tablespoon Olive Oil Extra Virgin

1/2 Teaspoon Turmeric

1 Teaspoon Dried Basil

1/2 Teaspoon Pink Himalayan Sea Salt

Half Teaspoon Dried Oregano

Instructions

Step 1.

Preheat oven to 350degF.

Step 2.

Add the cassava flour, salt and olive oil into a food processor and pulse for 30 seconds, until it forms crumbles.

Add the water and mix it at a low/dough setting until dough forms and is pulled off from its sides.

Step 3.

Preheat the skillet to medium-high.

Step 4:

Divide dough into 12 equal-sized balls.

Step 5:

With a tortilla press use a tortilla press to press each ball one at a on two pieces of paper.

Step 6:

Cook just one at one time in a heated pan for 30 seconds per side.

Cool on the cooling rack.

Continue for every tortilla.

Step 7:

Put the broth, as well as the cauliflower in a large pot and cover with a lid. Cook over medium heat, stirring frequently until the cauliflower is soft.

Step 8:

Remove the stove from heating by adding coconut milk. Blend until smooth.

Step 9:

Add the other ingredients for sauce to the pan and cook on medium heat until the sauce is boiling.

Reduce heat while cooking shrimp.

Step 10.

Incorporate olive oil into the skillet and cook until medium.

Step 11:

Sauté onions in the oil until they begin to caramelize.

Add the shrimp and seasonings.

Cook until the shrimp is cooked to your liking but be careful not to overcook.

Step 12:

Line a 9x13 baking dish with parchment.

Step 13:

Place the shrimp mix in each tortilla and roll up.

Place seam-side down into pan. If not, the tortillas won't be able to stay shut. Sprinkle sauce over chimichangas in an even layer

Step 14:

Bake in a preheated oven in the oven for about 10 minutes. Let it cool for 10 minutes before you enjoy! !

https://theautoimmuneinsomniac.com/2018/08/03/shrimp-chimichangas/

Crispy Wings & Sweet Potato Fries

AuthorName: Jaime Hartman

Ingredients

2 pounds of chicken wings

1. Teaspoon Grains-Free Baking Powder

Salt

1 teaspoon Garlic powder

1. Teaspoon Onion Powder

1. Teaspoon Dried Dill

1. Teaspoon Dried Thyme

2 Large Sweet Potatoes

2 Tablespoons of Melted Coconut Oil

Instructions

Step 1.

Heat oven to 375 degrees F.

Step 2.

In a bowl Mix baking powder 1 teaspoon salt onion powder, garlic powder, dill, and thyme.

Step 3.

Place the wings pieces in the large Ziplock bag. Mix baking soda and the seasoning mix and shake vigorously to ensure you're thoroughly coated.

Step 4:

Set up an oven. The wing pieces should be placed in the wire rack, spreading them to ensure that the wings aren't touching one another.

Step 5:

Bake in a rack made of wire on a baking tray, located near the center in the oven. Cook for about 40 mins.

Step 6:

Cut the sweet potato into pieces if you wish and cut them into fry-shaped pieces. Cut them in the closest size as you can. In this way, they cook evenly.

Step 7:

Pour them into coconut oil, then place them on a separate baking sheet. Put this baking sheet in the oven on the rack beneath the wings.

Step 8:

Add the sweet potatoes that you have prepared in the oven for 15 minutes after you have cooked the wings.

Step 9:

In the 40th minute, take out the sweet potato fries after 40 minutes. The oven should be set to 425 degrees.

Step 10.

In 10 mins, you can remove from the oven, then flip over with spatulas and then return in the oven to bake for an additional 10 minutes for them to be crisp on the opposite side. Put the sweet potatoes to the oven and allow them to roast. Be sure to watch the sweet potatoes and the wings to ensure to ensure they don't burn. Remove them once they have browned.

Serve with your favorite dip sauce.

Avocado and Shrimp Salad

Ingredients

For Cilantro Dressing/Marinade:

3. Tablespoon Fresh Lime Juice

Two Tablespoons Extra Virgin Olive Oil

1/2 Cup Fresh Cilantro, Chopped

Add Salt to Taste, and Pinch it.

Salad:

1 Pound Cooked Shrimp Deveined and Tail removed

2 Ripe Avocados

4 Cups Lettuce , or Baby Greens

Instructions

Mix the ingredients for the cilantro dressing or marinade dressing in a bowl, and mix.

Serve the dressing or marinade with cilantro on the inquisitive shrimp (make sure that any excess water is removed when using frozen shrimp that have been thawed. frozen shrimp). Mix to coat. Cover and chill for at least one an hour (2 or 3 is preferred).

Clean and dry the lettuce. Divide the lettuce among plates.

Cut avocado into bite-size wedges. Mix with lettuce.

Serve with marinated shrimp and any dressing leftover. Enjoy!

AIP chicken Lettuce Wraps Recipe

INGREDIENTS

2 Tablespoons Avocado Oil

2. Oz Mushrooms, Finely Chopped

Two Cloves of Garlic, Peeled and Minced

1 Small Piece of Ginger Minced and Peeled

9 Oz Ground Chicken

1. Teaspoon Lemon Juice

2 Tablespoons Coconut Aminos

4 Large Iceberg Lettuce Leaves

1 Spring Onion Finely Cut

Cilantro, To Garnish

INSTRUCTIONS

The avocado oil is heated in a skillet and sauté the mushrooms until golden.

Add the ginger, garlic and chicken ground and sauté till the meat is tender. Add the juice of a lemon as well as coconut aminos. Take the pan off the flame.

Pour the mix into large leaves of lettuce, and then sprinkle on the spring onions and the cilantro. Cover the leaves with a plate.

https://healingautoimmune.com/aip-chicken-lettuce-wraps-recipe

AIP Waldorf Salad

INGREDIENTS

2. Tablespoons Coconut Cream

1. Teaspoon Lemon Juice

Salt to Taste

1. Granny Smith or Another Green Apple Thinly Sliced

1. Stalk of Celery, Thinly Cut at An Angle

10. Grapes, Halved

One Head of Romaine Lettuce, chopped

INSTRUCTIONS

Prepare your AIP salad dressing mixing coconut cream with lemon juice. Add salt as needed.

Mix the dressing with the other ingredients, and toss until it is completely coated.

https://healingautoimmune.com/aip-waldorf-salad-recipe

AIP Italian Burgers Recipe

INGREDIENTS

1Pound Of Grass-Fed Ground Beef

Two Tablespoons Italian Seasoning

2 Tablespoons Garlic Powder

1 Tablespoon Onion Powder

INSTRUCTIONS

Blend all of the ingredients thoroughly before forming patties of burgers from the mix.

Grill or pan-fry coconut oil until it is done.

Chicken Salad Recipe using Grapes, Apple, And Celery

INGREDIENTS

1 Breast of Chicken, diced

Coconut Oil to cook chicken

25 grapes Halved

1 1/2 Gala Apple, Diced

1. Stalk of Celery, Diced

1/4 Cup Coconut Milk

Salt to Taste

INSTRUCTIONS

The chicken breasts that have been diced with coconut oil till it is cooked.

Let the chicken cool, then add the diced grapes, halved grapes, apple, and chopped celery in the large bowl. Mix in coconut milk, and season with salt to your preference.

Mix thoroughly.

5 Ingredient Salmon Patties

From Amanda Torres @ The Curious Coconut

INGREDIENTS

1. 14.75oz can of Wild Alaskan Pink Salmon

1/4 Cup + 2 Tbs of Canned Pumpkin

2. Tablespoon Coconut Flour

2 to 2 To Tablespoon Tapioca Starch

6. Tablespoon Pesto of Your Choice

Coconut Oil for Sauteing

INSTRUCTIONS

Step 1.

Take the salmon out of the can and then add the salmon into in a bowl. Remove bones

Step 2.

Mix the remaining ingredients in a bowl, along with salmon, and mix thoroughly.

Step 3.

The coconut oil can be heated in a large-sized fry pan for around 2 minutes.

Step 4:

Split the mixture of meat into eight sections. Make each section into a ball with your hands, then flatten it to form a patty.

Step 5:

The patties should be carefully placed in your hot pan. Cook for about 3-5 minutes on each side, until brown and crisped.

Don't flip them too soon. They are fragile patties, and can break If you flip them too quickly.

DINNER RECIPES

Nomato Sauce

via: Little Bites of Beauty

INGREDIENTS

1/4 Kabocha Squash, Peeled and Cut into Small Cubes

3 Carrots, cut into smaller cubes

1/2 Red Beet cut into smaller cubes

1 1/2 Teaspoons Olive Oil

1/3 Yellow Onion, Finely Chop

1. Clove Garlic Minced

5 Leaves Fresh Sage

Finely chopped1 Tablespoon Capers (Optional)

1 Tablespoon Dry Italian Herbs

1 Pinch Himalayan Salt To Taste

12 Cup Water, Or More If Required

1/2 Lemon Juiced

5 Leaves Fresh Basil, Chopped

INSTRUCTIONS

Step 1.

Mix kabocha squashand carrots and beets using a food processor. blend until coarsely grated.

Step 2.

In an oven over medium-high heat until it is it is hot. Add garlic, onion, and sage. Cook for around 1 minute. Add grated kabocha pumpkin as well as capers (if you wish), Italian herbs, and salt.

Step 3.

Add water to the saucepan. Cover and cook sauce with additional water, if necessary, until the Kabocha squash is soft, which takes about 30 minutes.

Step 4:

Mash the sauce with a fork to smoothen the sauce.

Step 5:

Mix the basil and lemon juice into the sauce, and let flavors mix.

Apple Fennel Casserole served with the Coconut-Turmeric twist

via: Little Bites of Beauty

INGREDIENTS

1. Teaspoon Olive Oil

2 Large Fennel Bulbs, Halved Crosswise

2. Teaspoons Ground Turmeric

3 Carrots Grated

1/2 Apple thinly cut

1/4 Cup Coconut Milk

INSTRUCTIONS

Step 1.

Preheat the oven to 380 degrees F. Grease a casserole dish with olive oil.

Step 2.

Put fennel pieces in the casserole dish. Dust their surface with turmeric. Cover them with apple and carrots. Pour coconut milk on the top.

Step 3.

The oven should be heated until tender, around 20 minutes. Flip the fennel halves over and mix. Place the dish in a casserole with foil and bake until the vegetables are tender, approximately 20 minutes.

Savory Sweet Potato Fries

by Carolyn Vaught

INGREDIENTS

2 large sweet potatoes, Peeled and cut into French Fry-Size pieces

1 Tablespoon Olive oil, or as required

2 Tablespoons Fresh Minced Rosemary,

Coarse Sea Salt

INSTRUCTIONS

Step 1.

Preheat oven until 425° F (220 ° C).

Step 2.

Mix the sweet potato, olive oil rosemary pepper, salt and olive oil in an enormous bowl until all ingredients are covered.

Step 3.

Place sweet potatoes on baking sheets.

Step 4:

In the oven, bake until the vegetables are tender for 20-30 minutes.

Coconut Crusted Taro Fries

By: Little Bites of Beauty

INGREDIENTS

1 Large Taro Root

1 Tablespoon Coconut Oil, Melted

2. Tablespoon Coconut Milk

1. Tablespoon Coconut Flakes

1 Pinch Himalayan Salt

INSTRUCTIONS

Step 1.

The oven should be preheated until it reaches 400 F.

Step 2.

Peel the taro root off and cut it into thin strips.

Step 3.

In a dish, make a mixture of coconut oil and milk and salt. Mix the taro strips with the mix. It may appear to be an excessive amount of liquid but the taro absorbs it.

Step 4:

Put the taro strips on a cookie sheet. sprinkle coconut flakes over top , then mix them well using your hands.

Step 5:

The baking time is 15 minutes. Then turn the fries around and bake for another 15 minutes. After 15 minutes, the coconut coating turns crispy and golden.

Roast Chicken with Rosemary

By LILQUIZ

INGREDIENTS

1. (3 12 lbs) Complete Chicken Dried

Salt to Taste

1 Small Onion quartered

1/4 Cup Fresh Rosemary Chopped

INSTRUCTIONS

Step 1

Bake at 350 degrees F.

Step 2

Sprinkle the chicken by adding salt, pepper and according to your liking. Fill it with rosemary and onion. Place chicken in a 9x13 inch baking dish or roasting dish.

Step 3.

Roast in the oven preheated in the oven for between 2 and 2 1/2 hours or until the chicken is cooked through and the juices flow clear. The cooking time can differ a bit based how large the chicken.

Easy Roasted Broccoli

By the name of karenatlincoln

INGREDIENTS

14 Ounces Broccoli

1 Tablespoon Olive Oil

Salt

INSTRUCTIONS

Step 1

Bake at 400°F until ready. F.

Step 2

Cut off the broccoli florets off the stalk. Peel the stalk and cut it into 1/4-inch-thick slices. Combine the stem and florets and olive oil together in a dish. place on a baking sheet to be sprinkled with salt.

Step 3.

Bake at the stove until the broccoli becomes tender, and uniformly brown in about 18 minutes.

https://www.allrecipes.com/recipe/240438/easy-roasted-broccoli/

Easy Grilled Chops of Lamb

by Noor

1 Cup White Vinegar Distilled

2 Teaspoons Salt

1 Tablespoon Minced Garlic

1 Onion, thinly cut

2 Tablespoons Olive Oil

2 Pounds Lamb Chops

INSTRUCTIONS

Step 1.

Mix the vinegar salt, garlic, onion, olive oil, and salt in a large bag that can be sealed until the salt is completely dissolving.

Step 2.

Add lamb, mix until coated, then allow to marinate in the refrigerator for two hours.

Step 3.

Grills can be heated up outdoors for medium-high temperatures.

Step 4:

Remove the lamb from marinade. Leave behind any onions that adhere onto the meat. Discard any marinade that remains.

Step 5:

Cover the exposed bones' ends by wrapping them in aluminum foil. This will stop their bones safe from burning.

Step 6:

Grill to your preferred degree of degree of doneness, around 3 minutes for medium. The chops are also able to be baked in the oven for broiled for about 5 minutes each portion for medium.

https://www.allrecipes.com/recipe/137917/simpl e-grilled-lamb-chops/?internalSource=streams&referringId=167 05&referringContentType=Recipe%20Hub&clickId =st_trending_b

Apple Pork Medallions

By: Wendi Washington-Hunt

INGREDIENTS

2-3 Cups of Sliced and Peeled 2 to 3 Cups Peeled and Sliced Fuji Apples (Sliced to 1/8 " Thick)

1 Teaspoon Cinnamon

1 Teaspoon Plus 1 Teaspoon Salt

2 Tablespoons Honey

2 Tablespoons Apple Cider Vinegar

1 Cup of Arrowroot Starch / Foul

1. Teaspoon Onion Powder

Half Teaspoon Garlic Powder

Two Tablespoons of Extra Virgin Olive Oil

1 pound Pork Loin/Tenderloin. Cut into 1/2 " Medallions

2 Teaspoons Fresh Thyme Leaves

INSTRUCTIONS

Step 1.

Within a bowl large enough, mix the apples, cinnamon and 1/2 teaspoon salt as well as honey and vinegar. Reserve.

Step 2.

A smaller container mix together arrowroot starch/flour 1 teaspoon salt, powdered onion as well as garlic powder.

Step 3.

Set the olive oil into a pan that is heated to medium-high. Once oil is heated to a simmer, dip the medallions of pork in the flour mixture, shaking off any excess, and then add the pan. Brown the medallions on both sides at a time, turning them over only once.

Step 4:

Reduce the heat to low to medium. Add the apple mixture and leaves of thyme to the pan. Cover then cook it for about 20 mins. Be sure to check frequently to ensure that the food does not get burned.

https://autoimmunewellness.com/apple-pork-medallions/

Moroccan Apricot Chicken

Written by Mickey Trescott

INGREDIENTS

1 Tablespoon Cooking Fat Solid

2 Onions, cut into large Chunks

4. Cloves Garlic Minced

1" Piece Ginger Peeled and Minced

2 Tablespoons Bone or water Broth

1. Teaspoon Sea Salt

1/2 Teaspoon Turmeric

2 Cups of chopped parsnips or Turnips

5 Cups of Butternut Squash Chopped (About One Small)

1/2 Cup Dried Apricots, Quartered

Half Cup Kalamata Olives, Pitted

1 1/2 lemon, juice, and Zest Reserved

2 pounds Boneless, Skinless Chicken Thighs

Cilantro along with Cauliflower Rice To Serve

INSTRUCTIONS

Step 1.

Pour the cooking fat to the bottom of the Instant Pot and then press on the "saute" button. Once the fat is been melted and the pan is hot and hot, add the onions and cook stirring for 7 minutes or until they are lightly brown. Add the ginger and garlic then cook stirring for about 30 seconds. Remove the pan from the flame.

Step 2.

Add the salt, water as well as turmeric, to the pan, and stir to mix. In the pot, add the vegetables for the root squash, apricots and squash citrus juice, olives and zest. Stir to mix. Incorporate the chicken thighs, and then place them within the vegetables. Close and secure the lid. Cook at "manual High tension" to cook for nine minutes.

Step 3.

If the timer is set to go off then utilize to use the "quick release" method to release the pressure using a an abrasive towel.

Serve over white rice made of cauliflower (or vegetable spirals) served by fresh chopped cilantro.

https://autoimmunewellness.com/instant-pot-moroccan-apricot-chicken/

Baked Stuffed Pumpkin with Balsamic Beef

from: Jo Romero

Ingredients

1 Large Whole Pumpkin

4 Slices Smoked Streaky Bacon

1. Red Onion cut and peeled.

1 . Large clove of Garlic Chopped, Peeled and Chopped

Large Handful Fresh Parsley Leaves, Chopped

1. Teaspoon Dried Sage

1 Pound Ground Beef

Splash - Around a Tablespoon Good Balsamic Vinegar

A Pinch of Salt

Instructions

Step 1.

prepare your oven for 400 degrees. Prepare a baking tray by covering it by aluminum foil. Place the tray aside

Step 2.

Clean the pumpkin and dry it. By using a razor blade carefully remove part of the pumpkin's top.

Cut off the 'lid' leaving a small opening enough for you to reach into. Take out all seeds and fibrous pieces.

Step 3.

Cut the bacon into pieces and cook it lightly in a large fry pan. When the bacon begins to crisp and brown and crisp, add the garlic, red onion parsley leaves, sage. Cook until the onion becomes translucent, which takes about 5-7 minutes.

Step 4:

Once the onion has become translucent then add the ground beef to the pan and cook, breaking the meat while cooking. Continue cooking for an additional 5 to 7 minutes, until the meat is cooked. Add a little bit of balsamic vinegar, one pinch of salt. Switch off the flame.

Step 5:

Utilizing a spoon with a slotted handle use a spoon to pour the cooked meat mixture in the pumpkin and press it into the pumpkin to fill it as much as you can, however, leave enough room at the top for you to place the pumpkin's lid over the top.

Step 6:

Put the stuffed pumpkin in the oven to cook for 45-50 minutes to ensure that the pumpkin remains soft and hot. Utilizing a spoon or spatula to gently press the lid of the pumpkin

Step 7:

Place the pumpkin on an unassuming plate or bowl to soak up the juices. Be cautious - it's hot and heavy! Cut off the pieces to serve each person, and top with a bit of extra meat that spills out when you serve.

https://www.comfortbites.co.uk/2015/10/roasted-stuffed-pumpkin-with-balsamic.html

Cassava Gnocchi

By: Julie Hunter

INGREDIENTS

3/4 Cup cooked/boiled Whole Cassava

12 Cup Otto's Cassava Flaour

3/4 Teaspoon Sea Salt

1.5 Tb Olive Oil

Salted water for boiling and oil to cook with

Further Olive Oil, Sea Salt and Rosemary Parsley along with Cauliflower Cheese to finish

INSTRUCTIONS

Step 1.

Prepare salted water pot to a rolling boil.

Step 2.

Blend cooked cassava in an immersion blender or food processor and then add flour as well as salt and oil and mix well until a smooth dough is formed.

Step 3.

Then cut it into the gnocchi

Step 4:

Cook gnocchi in two batches in water that is boiling. Gnocchi are cooked when they have risen at the top in about two minutes. Scoop them up and then drain them in a colander.

Step 5:

Cook gnocchi boiled in oil in a non-stick saute pan until desired hue.

Step 6:

Plate, and then finish with olive oil sea salt, fresh herbs (rosemary) as well as grated cheese from cauliflower.

http://www.flashfictionkitchen.com/cassava-gnocchi-paleo-aip-vegan/

Baked Prosciutto Wrapped, Chicken Saltimbocca

by: MICHELLE

Ingredients

1.5Pound 1 pound Chicken Breast (About three Chicken Breasts)

1/4-1/3 Teaspoon Salt

6-9 slices of Prosciutto

3 Tablespoon Avocado Oil

2. Tablespoon Olive Oil

2. Cloves Garlic Minced

3-4 Fresh Sage Leaves

Juice From 1/2 a Fresh Lemon

INSTRUCTIONS

Step 1.

Preheat the oven at 415 F and cover a baking dish by using parchment. Put aside.

Step 2.

Season lightly the chicken breast and wrap it in 2 pieces of prosciutto. Sprinkle the chicken with more seasoning.

Step 3.

Place your chicken into the dish, and sprinkle it with avocado oil, salt.

Step 4:

In the oven, bake for about 30 minutes , or till the prosciutto becomes crisp and the chicken has with an internal temperature of 160 F.

Step 5:

Remove the baking dish from the oven and place the baking dish aside.

Utilizing a small skillet in which you can warm the olive oil over a low temperatures.

Add the garlic to the pan and gently sauté until it becomes it is tender.

Incorporate the sage leaves in your pan, and allow to cook for about 1-2 minutes per side until you can lightly crisp the sage leaves.

Step 6:

Pour the garlic, olive oil and sage on the chicken, and then top it off with lemon juice. Serve warm.

https://unboundwellness.com/baked-prosciutto-wrapped-chicken-saltimbocca/?utm_source=Unbound+Wellness&utm_campaign=d5e7244409-EMAIL_CAMPAIGN_2019_05_22_05_02&utm_medium=email&utm_term=0_f6b7e1b9d7-d5e7244409-218476753

Salmon Tourtiere

written by the Dr. Sarah Ballantyne

INGREDIENTS

1 batch Perfect Pie Crust

Three large green plantains

3 cups Chicken Broth

3. Tablespoons Olive Oil

1 Medium Onion, Diced

1/2 Teaspoon Salt and More to Taste

1 teaspoon Savory or Thyme

1. Clove Garlic Minced

2 cans 15-ounces each of Salmon

INSTRUCTIONS

Step 1.

Prepare the Perfect Pie Crust (AIP). Refrigerate the dough till you're ready for rolling it.

Step 2.

Peel the plantains, then cut them to 1-1/2" chunks. Bring the broth to a rolling boil in medium-sized saucepot, over medium-high temperature. Add the plantains and simmer, with the lid off, until the plantain is soft, around 15 minutes.

Step 3.

In the meantime you heat olive oil over medium-high temperature in a small saucepan. Add onion , and stir frequently until the onion is browned, approximately 8 minutes.

Step 4:

Remove plantains from the stove and drain them, then set aside the liquid! Mash the plantains by hand using the fork or potato masherbefore returning the broth to where it appears to have the consistency of potatoes

Step 5:

Add salt to the plantains. Check the seasoning and adjust as needed. Include flavorful (or the herb thyme) as well as minced garlic.

Step 6:

Take out both salmon cans. Utilizing a fork, mix with the plantain mix. Keep the chunks of salmon as well as plantain , and do not to make it too smooth .

Step 7:

Bake at 375F until ready.

Step 8:

Make your dish. If making a meat pie, use a 9" deep-dish pie plate. If you're making a pot-pie or a pot pie, use an eight" or 9" casserole dish is ideal. The pie crust should be rolled out. If you are making a meat pie put a bottom layer on the bottom of your pie plate.

Step 9:

Mix the salmon and other ingredients into the dish, spreading it out to fill the dish uniformly. Put the pie crust gently over the top. Make sure you cut a few holes in the crust to allow for venting.

Step 10.

The baking time is 45 minutes, or until the crust begins to turn get brown. Take it out of the baking pan and enjoy!

https://www.thepaleomom.com/salmon-tourtiere-meat-pie/

SLOW COOKER RECIPES

Slow Cooker Braised Beef Slow Cooker

from Doctor. Amanda Paa

INGREDIENTS

1 1/2 to 2 Pounds from Beef Chuck Roast (Grass-Fed)

Two Tablespoons of Olive Oil Divided

3. Cloves Garlic, chopped and divided

1 1/4 Teaspoons Salt Divided

1 Teaspoon Dried Basil

1/2 Cup Chopped Leeks

15 olives (Any Kind)

1/4 Cup Water

1-pound carrots (cut the lengthwise in half and then cut them into 3-inch-long pieces)

4 fresh thyme sprigs

1/2 Tablespoon of arrowroot or tapioca starch (also called tapioca starch)

INSTRUCTIONS

Step 1.

Let the meat rest until it is at room temperature.

Step 2.

Mix 1 Tablespoon olive oil with 2 cloves of garlic 1 teaspoon salt and basil in one small bowl. Rub it over the roast. Cover it with a good coating. Mix it into the meat.

Step 3.

Set an iron skillet on high temperature. Incorporate one Tablespoon of oil and spread it over. Cook the meat for five minutes each side until the meat is browned.

Step 4:

Take the roast out. Add the remaining leeks and garlic. Cook on medium-high heat until the garlic is soft (about 4 minutes at a time). Transfer the stew into the Crockpot. Incorporate the remaining salt, carrots, olives and water and the thyme.

Step 5:

Place the the roast over the mixture of vegetables. Nestle it into it However, ensure that the roast is not touching the bottom of the cooker.

Step 6:

Cook at a low temperature for 5-6 hours, or until the dish is cooked.

Step 7:

After the roast is cooked thoroughly, take the roast from the oven and place it in a bowl to cool.

Step 8:

Sort the olives out of the mixture of carrots. Place the carrot mixture in separate bowl. Mash it using an potato fork or potato masher.

Step 9:

The drippings must be removed from the crockpot, and put them in a pan. The tapioca starch should be added the Drippings. Mix with a whisk, or fork, until the drippings are been thickened. If you need to, add water. It may be necessary the addition of salt.

Step 10.

Place the roast on the top of the mash of carrots. Cut the roast to the grain. Serve with the olives alongside.

https://heartbeetkitchen.com/2015/recipes/type/main-dish-recipes/slow-cooker-braised-beef-aip/

Nomato "Chili"

By Salixisme

INGREDIENTS

Four Cloves of Garlic, Crushed

2 medium onions, chopped

3 Cups Bone Broth

2lb Ground Beef (Grass-Fed)

Half Medium Rutabaga Peeled and Sliced

3 large Carrots Peeled and diced

1. Tablespoon Dried Oregano

2 medium beets, peeled and grated

1. Teaspoon Onion Powder

1. Teaspoon Dried Thyme

Half Teaspoon Garlic Powder

Half Teaspoon Ground Ginger

1/4 Teaspoon Ground Cloves

1/4 Teaspoon Cinnamon

Sea Salt to taste

2 Tablespoons Tapioca Flour to Thicken (Optional)

Drinking Water When Needed

Guacamole Homemade Guacamole to Serve

INSTRUCTIONS

Step 1.

Mix all ingredients in the crockpot , excluding the 2 tablespoons in tapioca meal. Mix well.

Step 2.

Cook at a low temperature until 8 hours.

Step 3.

Season according to your preference. If you want to thicken the chili by mixing tapioca flour with water.

Step 4:

Serve with a spoonful of homemade Guacamole. Serve.

Homemade Guacamole

INGREDIENTS

Two cloves garlic crushed

3 ripe avocados

2 Tablespoons avocado oil or 2 Tablespoons avocado oil

Juice and zest of 1 lime

Sea salt taste to your liking

INSTRUCTIONS

Mix all the ingredients in the food processor. Pulse until the mixture reaches that desired level of consistency.

https://salixisme.wordpress.com/2014/04/17/no mato-chilli-in-the-slow-cooker/

Slow Cooker Teriyaki Chicken

Michelle Hoover, NTP

INGREDIENTS

1 1.5 Pounds Chicken Breast 1.5 pounds of chicken breast

3/4 cup Coconut Aminos

2. Tablespoon Coconut Oil

2. Tablespoon Honey (Omit for Whole30)

1 Tablespoon Arrowroot Starch

1. Teaspoon Sea Salt

Three Tablespoons Fresh Orange Juice2 Teaspoon Fresh Ginger Grated

2. Teaspoon Onion Powder

3 Tablespoon Green Onion, Chopped

INSTRUCTIONS

Step 1.

With an electric whisk use a whisk to mix all the ingredients into a bowl, and put the bowl aside.

Step 2.

Place the chicken breasts into the Crockpot. Serve it with the sauce you prepared in step 1. Make sure you cover the chicken thoroughly.

Step 3.

Cook at low heat up to 8 hours.

Step 4:

Remove the chicken from the Crockpot. The chicken is shred with two forks. It is possible to slice it using a fork, if you prefer.

Step 5:

Pour the sauce on top of the chicken breasts. Serve it over your green onions. Enjoy it along with your preferred sides.

https://unboundwellness.com/slow-cooker-teriyaki-chicken/

The Slow Cooker Short Ribs Slow Cooker in Plum Sauce

By Tara Perillo

INGREDIENTS

3 Pounds Beef Short Ribs

1 Tablespoon Coconut Oil

2. Tablespoon Raw Honey

5 Plums Chopped, Pitted and Chopped

1/3 cup Coconut Aminos

2 cups organic Beef Broth

1. Tablespoon Crushed Garlic

1 Small Piece of Fresh Ginger, Peeled and Diced

1/2 Onion and Sliced Thin

1/8 Teaspoon Salt

1 Tablespoon Arrowroot Starch

4 Ounces of Large Mushrooms Cut into slices

INSTRUCTIONS

Step 1.

In a large pot cook the short ribs in a single side.

Step 2.

Mix all the ingredients remaining, with the exception of the mushrooms and the arrowroot in the crockpot.

Step 3.

Add the short ribs that have been browned to the crockpot and then put it in..

Step 4:

For 4 hours, cook. Then add the arrowroot and mushrooms to the crockpot.

Step 5:

Mix the ingredients. If it's not whisked enough, you will end up with lumps.

Step 6:

The cooking continues for an additional half an hour.

Step 7:

Serve the sauce with vegetables on top.

http://www.paleocajunlady.com/slow-cooker-short-ribs-in-plum-sauce-recipe/

Delicious Slow Cooker Chicken Lemon Creamy Kale Soup

By Jessica Flanigan

INGREDIENTS

Six Cups of Bone Broth Divided

4 cups of precooked, shredded Chicken (you may start by preparing two raw chicken breasts if you want)

1 Bunch Kale

Two Tablespoons of Fresh Lemon Juice

3 Lemons

12 Cup Olive Oil

1 cup Onions, Large onion

Salt to Taste

INSTRUCTIONS

Step 1.

Clean the leaves of kale thoroughly. Then, stack half of the leaves of kale. Slice into 1/2-inch pieces. Do the same thing with the remaining half. Set aside.

Step 2.

Place 2 cups of liquid bone broth along with olive oil and chopped onion into the blender. Blend until it is completely homogeneous (1 or 2 minutes).

Step 3.

Mix the ingredients from Step 2 along with the rest of the broth, the chicken that has been shredded the remaining lemon juice, kale, pinch of salt and the zest of all three lemons into the crockpot.

Step 4:

Cook at a low temperature for about 6 hours. Stir a few times.

https://jessicaflanigan.com/recipe/lemon-chicken-kale-soup/

Ham Slow Cooker (Paleo as well as AIP)

By: Michele Spring

INGREDIENTS

1 - 6 Pound Ham Roast

1/4 Cup Honey

12 Cup Orange Juice

2. Teaspoon Dried Rosemary

4. Tablespoon Coconut Oil

The Zest 1 Orange

1. Tablespoon Apple Cider Vinegar

INSTRUCTIONS

Step 1.

Place the ham in a slow cooker.

Step 2.

Include all the other ingredients to the ham.

Step 3.

Cook at a low temperature for 4-6 hours.

https://thrivingonpaleo.com/slow-cooker-ham-paleo-and-aip/

DESSERTor SNACK RECIPES

Halloween AIP Marshmallow Ghosts

By Dr. Sarah Ballantyne

INGREDIENTS

1 Cup of Mild-Flavored Honey

1 Cup Water, Divided

1/4 Cup Gelatin

1 Teaspoon Vanilla

Arrowroot Powder for Dusting

Dry Cranberries or Raisins to help with Mouth and eyes

INSTRUCTIONS

Step 1.

Make honey and half the boiling water within a pot to 240 °.

Step 2.

Bloom the gelatin that is in the second part of the pool.

Step 3.

Put the gelatin into the bottom of the standing mixer, and begin whipping while pouring the hot honey mixture on top and allow it to whip on medium-high for 10 to 12 minutes, until soft peaks appear.

Step 4:

Scoop marshmallows into a piping bag that has an a 1/2-inch round piping tip. Pipe the marshmallow mixture onto a baking sheet lined with parchment sprinkled with powdered arrowroot.

Step 5:

Moving quickly adding dried fruit, while the marshmallow remains sticky. Pipe up to 4-5 times and then add"eyes" and "mouth," then "eyes" along with the "mouth" before continuing pipe.

Step 6:

Make sure to sprinkle the marshmallows liberally with powdered arrowroot and let them sit for at least 4 hrs or for a night.

https://www.thepaleomom.com/halloween-aip-marshmallow-ghosts/

The Healing Pumpkin of Halloween Turmeric Gummies

by Michelle Hoover

INGREDIENTS

1 Cup Coconut Milk (Full Fat)

1 Cup Pumpkin Puree

1/4 Cup Gelatine that is fed by Grass Gelatin

1 Tablespoon Turmeric

1. Teaspoon Vanilla Extract (Alcohol-Free)

1 Tablespoon Honey in Raw Honey

1 Teaspoon Cinnamon

12 Teaspoon Pumpkin Pie Spice Blend (

INSTRUCTIONS

Step 1.

In a high-speed blender combine all the ingredients, excluding gelatin. Turn the blender on high until blended.

Step 2.

Pour the mix into a saucepan and cook on medium heat. Incorporate the gelatin a bit at a moment, constantly stirring to ensure there aren't any lumps. Continue it will be heating at medium temperature for approximately five minutes.

Step 3.

Remove from the heat and let cool.

Step 4:

Mix the ingredients in pumpkin molds and chill for at minimum an hour.

https://unboundwellness.com/healing-halloween-pumpkin-turmeric-gummies-aip-Paleo/

Fudgy Brownies from Collagen

INGREDIENTS

2/3 Cup Plantain Flour

2/3 cup Carob Powder

2. Tablespoon Carob Powder

7 Tablespoon Collagen Peptides

1/2 Teaspoon Salt

1. Teaspoon Baking Soda

Two Small Bananas Mashed

Six Tablespoons Maple Syrup

1/4 Cup Coconut Oil Melted

2. Teaspoon Vanilla Extract

INSTRUCTIONS

Step 1.

Grease an 8x8 baking dish.

Step 2.

Mix dry ingredients together in a bowl, using an electric whisk.

Step 3.

Incorporate wet ingredients into the bowl and stir to mix well and make sure that the dry ingredients are moistened.

Step 4:

Utilizing a hand mixer mix until the entire mixture is combined and you no longer see chunks of banana.

Step 5:

Pour the batter into greased 8x8 dish, then smooth across the top to expose the edges.

Step 6:

Bake at 375 degrees for 25 to 28 minutes.

Step 7:

Let let it completely cool. Keep in the refrigerator.
**

https://rallypure.com/fudgy-collagen-brownies-aip-paleo-gluten-free/

Minty Thins

by Wendi's AIP Kitchen

INGREDIENTS

The cookie component:

1/2 C. Cassava Flour

1/4 C. Arrowroot Starch/Flour

1/8 C. Carob Powder

1. T. Gelatin

1 2. Baking Soda

1/2 C. Palm Shortening

Half C. Coconut Sugar

1 T. Pure Peppermint Oil

5T. Water

The frosting is:

2. T. Pure Maple Syrup

2. T. Carob Powder

131

1 . T. Water

1/8 C. Coconut Oil

2. T. Coconut Butter

1 T. Pure Peppermint Oil

Five T. Hot Water

INSTRUCTIONS

Step 1.

Preheat oven to 350 degrees F. Within a large bowl delicately mix together the cassava flour carob, arrowroot, gelatin and baking soda. Put aside.

Step 2.

In a mixing bowl, cream shortening. Add sugar, and then cream again. Add peppermint oil and then cream one more time.

Step 3.

By hand, mix in dry ingredients. Then , mix in water, one teaspoon at a moment, until it reaches an consistency that is similar to wet sand. It appears dry and fragile, but if you take a few slivers of it, it will stick to itself.

Step 4:

Collect the dough. Make a half-portion of the dough and roll it into an oblong. Then, roll it between two sheets of parchment paper with a thickness of 1/8"-1/4". The parchment should be removed from the top.

Step 5:

With 1-inch and a 2-inch cutter make shapes and then place these on the greased baking sheet. Baking for about 10 minutes. Repeat the process with the remainder of the dough. Allow to cool.

Step 6:

Create the frosting! In a small mixing bowl, mix sugar syrup with carob powder, and 1 tablespoon water.

Step 7:

In an glass measuring cup, slowly melt the coconut butter and coconut oil. Don't overheat! Place in the microwave for 10 seconds at a time. Stir. Perhaps do 10 seconds, then stir.

Step 8:

Slowly whisk the melted blend into carob mix in small increments at one time. Continue to whisk, and then add 1 teaspoon in peppermint oil.

Continuously whisking, add hot water, one teaspoonful at one time.

Step 9:

Each time take a dip on the top of cookies , then place them on cooling racks. Put a cookie sheet underneath the rack in order to catch the drips. Allow the cookies to set. Cool them down to set the frosting!

https://wendisaipkitchen.com/2019/02/07/minty -thins-aip-paleo/#wpzoom-recipe-card

Paleo AIP Blueberry Cheesecake

By Ambra Torelli

INGREDIENTS

for the Crust:

1/4 Cup of unsweetened coconut shredded

1/4 Cup Tigernut Flour

1 teaspoon Carob Powder

1 Teaspoon Vanilla Extract

1 Teaspoon Cinnamon Powder

4 . Dried Apricots About

1 Tablespoon coconut butter

1 Tablespoon Coconut Oil Room Temperature

1 Tablespoon 1 Tablespoon Lemon Juice

To make for the Cheesecake Filling:

1 Cup Fresh Blueberries

1/4 Cup Frozen Strawberries

2. Tablespoon Coconut Flour

1 Tablespoon 1 Tablespoon Lemon Juice

1 Tablespoon + 1/2 Teaspoon Collagen

5/8 Cup Coconut Yogurt

1/8 Cup Coconut Milk

Half Teaspoon Vanilla Extract

2 1/2 Teaspoon Gelatin Powder

To decorate:

1/4 cup Raspberries One Small Handful

1. Teaspoon Coconut Cream

1 Teaspoon Coconut Flakes that are unsweetened, chopped

INSTRUCTIONS

Step 1.

Mix strawberries, blueberries and lemon juice. Add collagen and coconut flour in the high-speed blender, and blend until it is smooth.

Step 2.

Transfer this mixture into a bowl, then mix in the coconut yogurt, and place aside.

Step 3.

Make the coconut milk and vanilla in a small saucepan and once it is hot (do not let it come to a point of boiling) remove it from the heat and mix in the gelatin powder and mix it thoroughly with the help of a milk mixer.

Step 4:

Incorporate the coconut milk to the blueberry mixtureand mix until well combined. Let the AIP cheesecake mixture cool at room temperature while you make the jam with raspberries.

Step 5:

Squash the raspberries, and cook them in a small pot for about 2 to 3 minutes until they've turned into a thick jam. Allow to cool within the fridge.

Step 6:

Mix all the ingredients with a food processor, then process until you get an attractive, crumbly mix.

Step 7:

Make the dough flat into the 6'' diameter silicon mold. Set it to rest in the fridge.

Step 8:

After the cheesecake's filling is at room temperature Pour it over the crust. Drizzle a few drops of raspberry jam and coconut cream over it, making swirls using the help of a toothpick.

Step 9:

Cool the Paleo AIP Blueberry Cheesecake for at most 1 1/2 hours. The filling will get thicker to the proper consistency!

https://www.littlebitesofbeauty.com/paleo-aip-blueberry-cheesecake/

Lemon Cake Cookies

By Bre'anna

INGREDIENTS

Cookies for the sake of cookies.

1/3 cup Coconut Flour

1/3 cup Arrowroot Flour

1 teaspoon cream of Tartar

3 Teaspoons Baking Soda

1/8 Teaspoon Sea Salt

1/8 Teaspoon Turmeric

1/4 Cup Freshly squeezed Lemon Juice

1 Tablespoon of Freshly Grated Lemon Zest

1/4 Cup Applesauce, At Room Temperature

1 Cup Coconut Butter Softened

2 Tablespoons Honey

2. 2 Tablespoons Coconut Oil

1. Teaspoon Vanilla Extract

1 Tbs. Gelatin

for the Icing

1/4 cup Arrowroot Flour

2 Tablespoons Honey

1 1/2 teaspoons lemon Juice

INSTRUCTIONS

Step 1.

Preheat oven to 325 degrees. Two cookie sheets should be lined using parchment.

Step 2.

Within a bowl stir together dried ingredients, including coconut flour salt, arrowroot flour baking soda.

Step 3.

Mix together the applesauce, coconut butter lemon zest lemon juice honey, coconut oil, honey and vanilla.

Step 4:

Prepare gelatin egg substitute: Whisk 1 tablespoon gelatin into 1 tablespoon lukewarm water. Add 2 tablespoons of boiling water. Stir vigorously until the water is completely dissolving and foamy.

Step 5:

Mix gelatin egg substitute into the stand mixer. Beat until combined.

Step 6:

Incorporate dry ingredients into a the stand mixer, and mix on medium until combined.

Step 7:

Utilizing a tablespoon to scoop dough out, drop it on cookie sheets. Make each cookie flat using one of the cups, to create 1 1/2 to 2" circles.

Step 8:

Bake for 18-23 minutes or until the cookies have a golden brown appearance around the edges and slightly soft to the feel. Cool completely on a wire rack.

Step 9:

To make the icing, whisk all ingredients of icing together. Sprinkle the icing on tops of the cooled cookies.

Cover and store at room temperature in order to make soft biscuits, or store in the refrigerator for more firm cookies.

http://empoweredsustenance.com/paleo-lemon-cookies/

Paleo Triple Berry

by Joanna Smith

INGREDIENTS

2 Cups Fresh Strawberries, Sliced

2 Cups Fresh Blueberries

2 Cups of fresh Blackberries

To make the Cake:

1.5 Cups Arrowroot Starch

1 Cup Coconut Flour

2. Teaspoons Baking Soda

2 Tablespoons of Cream of Tartar

1/2 Teaspoon Salt

1/2 Cup Coconut Oil, Melted

1-14 Ounce Coconut Milk that is Full-Fat

1/2 Cup Applesauce

1/3 Cup Raw Honey

1 Tablespoon 1 Tablespoon Lemon Juice

To make Coconut Whipped Cream: Coconut
Whipped Cream:

3- 14-Ounce Cans Coconut Cream)

5-6 Tablespoons Maple Syrup

for the Berry Compote (Optional)

2 Cups Frozen Mixed Berries

2 Tablespoons Maple Syrup or Honey

1. Tablespoons Lemon Juice

1. Teaspoon Arrowroot Starch

INSTRUCTIONS

Step 1.

Preheat oven to 350°F. Grease the 9x13 cake pan with a '.

Step 2.

Clean and prepare the for berries. Set aside.

Step 3.

Combine dry ingredients for the cake in large bowls. Mix wet ingredients except lemon juice in a smaller bowl. Add wet ingredients to dry ingredients and mix. Mix in lemon juice and stir until the lemon juice is fully incorporated.

Step 4:

Place cake batter in the pan. Bake for 20-25 minutesor until toothpicks come out clear. Cool.

Step 5:

While the cake is baking while cake is baking, whip the coconut cream with a stand mixer . Then, slowly introduce the maple syrup one tablespoon at a time. Put the cake at room temperature until it is ready to use.

Step 6:

In a small pot on medium-low heat, cook frozen frozen fruits, honey as well as lemon juice, for approximately 8-10 minutes while stirring often. After the berries are broken down and the mixture is bubbly, mix in the Arrowroot starch and cook for another 2 to 3 minutes. Take off the heat and let cool.

Step 7:

Cut the cake after cooling into tiny squares (I created six rows across and 8 vertically). The first two rows of cake to the top of the trifle bowl.

Step 8:

The cake can be topped by adding 1/3 coconut-whipped cream. Add 1/3 of the fresh fruit followed by half of the Compote of berries.

Step 9:

Repeat the layers, leaving one piece of fresh fruit for the top. Finish the trifle by adding one last layer of cake, and the rest of the whip cream. (You'll have a few portions of cake left however it's not a problem!)

Step 10.

Cover the top portion of trifle using the reserved berries. Cover it with plastic. Refrigerate until you are ready to serve.

https://fedandfulfilled.com/paleo-triple-berry-trifle/

Soft Pretzel Bites

by: Heather Resler

INGREDIENTS

Pure Maple Syrup 2 Tablespoons

Extra Virgin Olive Oil - 3 Tablespoons

1/2 Cup Full-Fat Coconut Milk

2 Tablespoons Puree of Pumpkin Puree

Cassava Flour - 1 Cup

1 Teaspoon baking soda

2. Tablespoons Coconut Flour

Salt 1/2 Teaspoon

Water - 1 to 1-1/2 Quarts

Baking Soda 3 Tablespoons

Coarse Salt - For Sprinkling

INSTRUCTIONS

Step 1.

Preheat oven to 375°F. grease a baking tray with some olive oil.

Step 2.

A mixing bowl mix oil, maple syrup coconut milk, pumpkin. Stir together.

Step 3.

Mix in the cassava flour coconut flour, baking soda and salt until you have the dough into a fine, smooth consistency.

Step 4:

Create in a 3/4-inch length and then cut it into tiny pretzel bites.

Step 5:

The baking soda until they reach a boil in a medium saucepan. Inject some pretzel pieces and allow to simmer until it is 30 seconds. Take the bites out with a spoon and transfer to the baking sheet. Repeat with the remaining.

Sprinkle salt on top.

Cook for about 30 mins.

Cool.

http://createdelicious.com/paleo-soft-pretzels-cassava-flour/

Guacamole

By Adrienne

INGREDIENTS

2 Avocados

1 Tablespoon Lime Juice

1 Teaspoon Salt

Half Miniature Red Onion (Chopped)

1/4 Cup Chopped Cilantro

2. Cloves Garlic (Minced)

INSTRUCTIONS

Step 1.

Place all the ingredients into the bowl.

Step 2.

Mix until combined.

https://wholenewmom.com/recipes/aip-guacamole-autoimmune-paleo-guacamole/

AIP Cheese (Dairy Free, Nut Free Soy Free)

Written by: Jaime Hartman

INGREDIENTS

1 Pound Butternut Squash Peeled and Cut (Frozen is great for storage)

Water

3 Tablespoons Avocado Oil

4 Tablespoons Gelatin

1 Cup Nutritional Yeast

1/3 Cup Tapioca Starch

1 1/2 Teaspoons Fine Sea Salt

INSTRUCTIONS

Step 1.

Put the squash along with about half one cup of water in a medium-sized saucepan. Bring to an unbeatable boil, then lower temperature and cover. Let it simmer until extremely soft (about 6 to 9 minutes).

Step 2.

Get rid of the water and dispose.

Step 3.

Transfer squash to a high-powered blender

Step 4:

Add the remaining ingredients to the mix. Blend until it is smooth.

Step 5:

Line the inside of a small loaf pan or another vessel with parchment, then put the mix in. The mixture should be spread as evenly as you can.

Step 6:

Place in the refrigerator and let it cool until the temperature is set (about about two hours).

https://gutsybynature.com/2017/03/19/aip-cheese-dairy-free-nut-free-soy-free/

Oven-Roasted Root Vegetable Chips (AIP)

Author: Jaime Hartman

INGREDIENTS

The root vegetables (such as sweet potatoes, etc.))

Oil (coconut oil is recommended)

The process of seasoning (AIP Paleo Powder is a great option)

INSTRUCTIONS

Step 1.

Preheat oven to 425 degrees.

Step 2.

Select the root vegetables you are planning to use, and then peel them and slice them in the thinst way you can.

Step 3.

For every pound of vegetable it will take around 1 tablespoon oil. If you're making use of coconut oil you'll require it to be melted first.

Step 4:

In the oil, and then distribute equally on the sheets of.

Step 5:

Lightly-seasonal.

Put in the oven to bake for 10 mins. After 10 minutes, the chips will begin to turn brown. Use tongs to flip the chips and move them around as much as you can. You can also remove chips that are near the desired level of crispness.

Step 6:

Return the pan to the oven and continue baking. Every two minutes, check the oven taking out the chips that have reached the desired crispness and returning the remainder in the oven. After 15 to 18 minutes, everything is completed.

Add a touch of seasoningas you like.

Serve them on the same day you prepare them.

https://gutsybynature.com/2019/04/02/oven-roasted-root-vegetable-chips-aip/

Herb & Garlic Crackers (Paleo, AIP)

By: Julie Hunter

INGREDIENTS

3/4 Cup Cassava Flour

1/4 Cup Tigernut Flour

1. Teaspoon Sea Salt

1. Tb Dry Herbs (Rosemary, Thyme, Oregano)

1 Tablespoon Garlic Powder

1/4 cup Coconut Oil

1/8 Cup Cold Water

INSTRUCTIONS

Step 1.

Preheat oven to 350 degrees Fahrenheit.

Step 2.

Mix the first five ingredients together.

Step 3.

Cut the coconut oil with an ice-cream maker until you are left with small pea-sized pieces of the mixture.

Step 4:

Add the water in small tablespoons until the dough is smooth and you are able to shape it into a smooth disc. Keep it in the fridge to chill for one hour (or put it into the freezer to chill for 20 minutes).

Step 5:

Roll up to about 1mm thickness. Then cut the cracker shapes of your choice and roll again as required until the mixture has been used to. Crackers should be finished with a scattering of herbs and salt.

Step 6:

Bake on a parchment-lined baking tray for 10 to 15 minutes, or until the crackers begin to get brown around the edges (keep an check on them, as they may burn easily the cooking time will vary depending on the oven).

http://www.flashfictionkitchen.com/herb-garlic-crackers-paleo-aip/

Chapter 5: Lifestyle Modifications To Comply With The Aip

"You should not focus on the reason the reasons why you aren't able to do something as the majority of people do. Instead, you should think about what you might be able to do and become one of the few exceptions." Steve Case Steve Case

I

It takes between about four or five years tests before one is finally given the diagnosis of an autoimmune disease. When they finally discover the cause of their suffering over the years, doctors are generally eager to use drugs against the autoimmune disease.

The most popular treatments include:

* Anti-rheumatic medications that alter the course of disease (DMARDs)

DMARDs have the potential to slow the progress of an autoimmune condition or prevent it from progressing in any way.

* Biologics

They are made from synthetic proteins, they are the newest class of DMARDs. TNF (TNF) blockers comprise the most prominent category of this treatment. TNFs lower the inflammatory proteins.

* Nonsteroidal anti-inflammatory medications (NSAIDs)

NSAIDs aid in reducing certain symptoms of autoimmune diseases , such as pain, swelling and stiffness.

* Corticosteroids

Prednisone is among the most frequently employed corticosteroid. It combats inflammation by reducing the body's immune system. Corticosteroids in high doses shouldn't be employed for long-term use due to severe adverse consequences.

*IVIg (intravenous immunoglobulin)

IVIg is administered via intravenously. It is made up of antibodies. It does not hinder the normal functions in the system of immunity, while helping it to get back to normal.

Treatments for medical conditions that could be added, based on the immune system. could include:

* Plasmapheresis

Through this process, plasma along with the bad antibodies, are removed in your blood. This process is used only in the most serious of cases since it can seriously affect the immune system.

* Surgery

It is not often required. The most common complications that require surgery are obstructions in the bowel (which can cause by the Crohn's illness) and joint injury (which can be caused by various types of arthritis).

Autoimmune conditions may affect your muscle to nerves, all the way to your organs that are vital, as there's no substitute for regular medical attention. However, as a supplement to your medical treatment you must make some lifestyle adjustments as well. These lifestyle changes could be so detrimental that you're able to completely go off any medication! All you have to do is find two reasons why your immune system is not in equilibrium and the best way to correct it.

The effects of autoimmune disease can be catastrophic. Some cause total disability. Certain cases even cause death. But, lifestyle modifications can aid those suffering from an autoimmune disorder to not just live a healthier life in general, but also to lessen the symptoms.

There is usually an origin of the inflammation. Finding the cause may provide an opportunity to live a better life. It could be due to food, dehydration, toxic burden, drugs, infection inactivity, poor sleep habits and stress.

Investigating the root of your discomfort is a process of trial and trial and. It takes time and perseverance. It's not easy, but it's worth the effort. Inflammation reduction can reduce the risk to develop an auto-immune condition or ailment, or bring you into Remission.

Take Dietary Guidelines for the Autoimmune Protocol Diet

We've covered this extensively however, this chapter would not be complete without a section that would emphasize how important eating a balanced diet is. The AIP is not only essential to reducing inflammation, and thus alleviating symptoms, but proper nutrition can boost the function of your immune system. Your doctor might have details about other changes in your diet that can help manage the specific autoimmune condition you suffer from.

Use supplements

As I discussed in chapter three, obtaining the correct nutrients and vitamins in your diet is crucial. In addition, taking probiotics, fish oils vitamin C, vitamin D may help to reduce the symptoms naturally, by calming the immune system. Quercetin, grapeseed extract and rutin are also anti-inflammatory properties.

Drink plenty of water

Ninety-two percent in our blood is composed of water. Our skin is made up of 64 percent water. The brain and the heart comprise 73 percent water. The muscles and kidneys of our bodies comprise 79% water. The lungs contain 83% water and our bones comprise 31 percent water. Therefore, not drinking enough water can cause problems with the bodily functions of your body and could result in long-term health problems. The process your body undergoes as it dehydrates causes inflammation throughout your body. Inflammation that is prolonged can lead to the development of autoimmune diseases. In addition, inflammation can trigger flare-ups and signs in people suffering from an autoimmune condition.

Reduce the Toxic Impact of Your Life

We are exposed to harmful chemicals all the time. Pesticides are present in the foods we eat and in the air we breathe, the chemicals found in our everyday products for hygiene we use, as well as chemical contaminants and other substances in the water we consume. They don't disappear! They are absorbed by our body.

Based on a study of five years conducted by The Centers of Disease Control conducted there are traces of 212 chemicals are found within your body! There could be additional substances that they haven't been tested for. A multitude of chemicals that directly impact our lives are utilized every day.

Researchers don't know the different risks are in all these chemical exposures yet. There's been very little of research conducted. It has been proven that the greater the burden of toxic substances more likely you are to develop an auto-immune disorder. Research has also shown that reducing your burden of toxic substances could slow down, stop or even reverse the effects of your immune system!

Chapter 6: Eating Out On The Autoimmune Protocol

" It is important to look for an individual to drink and eat with prior to looking for something to eat or drink." Epicurus Epicurus

A

Being a full-time, working mother One of the things that I love every single week is having dinner on Friday nights in the restaurant. It's a nice break from the frantic cooking and cleaning up after an eventful week. When I first began AIP I was disappointed to discover that dining out was not something I could enjoy. It was a daunting mission to find a place in my city that could be AIP conforming. Therefore, one of my favourite activities was taken away from me. After a while, I was annoyed to forfeit the weekly treat for surviving the hectic week. I decided to go out and attempt to have a healthy meal and make the best decision I could with what was on their menu. It was a complete catastrophe. I developed an autoimmune reaction in a couple of hours after eating. I went again unable to eat at restaurants and was very unhappy about it!

Dining Out

It's true that I'm not the only one. One of the most common reason people use to justify not taking AIP is the fact that they'll no longer be able dine out in the future. After some research I came across a method that works well for dining out. It requires a little time to plan, however you will still enjoy a meal with family and friends and still be on the AIP. There are some tricks to make this process easier. In this section, we're going to look at those techniques and also discuss eateries that offer AIP choices.

My first suggestion for regaining the freedom to dine out at restaurants is:

Research prior to making a decision.

If you are on a restricted diet due to allergies or an autoimmune disorder simply winging it and ordering off the normal menu once you arrive at the restaurant can be an unintentional disaster. Do yourself and the staff at the restaurant the favor of looking over the menu on their website prior to you leave. Select a variety of items that you think could be suitable for your diet, with a some minor changes. For instance, you could grill meat or salad.

When I looked over the food menu, I'd often make a call prior to. If I could, I would speak to the service staff and inquired about any concerns I had regarding the food preparation (such such as, is it prepared by using canola oil? Can I substitute it by olive oil, since there is a reaction to it in me? Are the steaks marinated?) making a reservation in advance meant I could get my meal reduced prior to my arrival there.

My next suggestion goes hand-in-hand with the final tip:

Do not be afraid to ask questions.

If you call ahead or ask for the waiter and the wait staff when you get there, you'll have to seek clarification regarding the menu. Particularly in the phase of elimination of AIP There are many common ingredients like black pepper for instance which you are not allowed to use. You must inquire whether these ingredients are included within the meals you are able to narrow down from their menu, and if they're possible to eliminate. For instance If they marinate of their meats in a sauce that has sugar as well as black pepper, you'll have to choose a different option like the grilled salmon that they don't marinade in and can be cooked in olive oil, but without pepper. Be courteous and polite when you ask questions. Be gentle and respectful. My grandmother always used to say, "You draw more flies by using honey than vinegar".

Another thing I have found useful is:

Choose the best restaurant.

Let's face it, some varieties of food are likely to being more AIP compatible than other. For instance, fresh Mediterranean types of food such as Greek and Lebanese will more often include dishes that fit into your AIP diet, compared to an French restaurant with many cream-based sauces and butter used in cooking items. Another restaurant type that I have found to be effective is vegetarian restaurants. I noticed that, generally that the staff in these were more willing to modify the menu items. Another good option was to try some Asian eateries like Thai.

My next suggestion is this:

You should be prepared to mix and match the menu.

The menu you choose may not be the best for you. For instance, let's suppose that the salmon that was grilled was served with rice as one of the dishes. Rice isn't allowed when you follow an AIP diet. Therefore, you should make a request to the restaurant to substitute it with a salad that has no croutons or tomatoes and without dressing. So, you can enjoy a complete meal, and you still adhere to your AIP diet.

Another thing I found useful was

Take your personal AIP approved salad dressing and other condiments.

162

Let's face it, finding AIP acceptable dressings and condiments that you love, takes some effort and trial and. I couldn't find any restaurant in my small town that offer these products that's not surprising. Lemon and olive oil as your sole dressing get tired quickly, or at least for me. Therefore, I put all of my most-loved dressings and condiments in containers for single-use use in my refrigerator. When I got to the door, I was able to easily grab them for work or to go to a restaurant.

Another useful trick is:

Simple is best.

I discovered that it's simpler and more secure to purchase easy, simple meals like grilling meat, sauteed vegetables and so on. The fewer ingredients you have the fewer ingredients, the more flavorful. Soups and casseroles contain multiple ingredients that they're almost guaranteed to contain something that is not AIP approved. I have found it simpler to avoid these dishes completely. My general rule of thumb when dining out is that the less complicated your meal, the more enjoyable.

I also discovered this to be useful:

Remain a loyal customer.

After I discovered a place that I could work with to become AIP conforming, I was a regular customer. I formed a rapport with the staff, and even prepared a list of the foods I could not eat at one restaurant where the chef requested it. It was a good idea to do this as it helped make the experience more enjoyable for all. I was confident that I could dine there. They were aware that I was a good client, who left a nice tip and will be returning.

The next point is in line with the first one:

Don't forget to tip generously.

I've spoken about these two things in a casual manner in other tips However, they are worth being repeated. The restaurant is asking you to go beyond. Don't be upset if you discover the meal options on the menu doesn't be a success. Be kind. Thank them for going above and beyond to accommodate you . Also, tip them well! Be sure to show your appreciation by giving them a tip. Write them a positive review on the internet. These actions will help to creating an unforgettable dining experience. What you get out of life is the things is put in it. If you show a bit of generosity and kindness and most of the time you will be greeted with kindness and compassion.

Once you've completed these tasks, head out with your buddies. Have fun, eat fantastic food, laugh and live. Do not let an autoimmune illness take these wonderful aspects of your life.

Food Delivery

I'm going to be honest with you here. The first time I attempted to follow AIP I returned to my usual eating routine in just two weeks. The protocol wasn't the reason why it didn't work. It wasn't that I needed to give up all kinds of food items. But the reason my "fell out of the loop" or so it was called was because I was unable to cook separate meals for me and my family each day. It just became too much. But then I found something that made the entire process manageable for me. This is the reason for my accomplishment: AIP meal delivery services.

It wasn't just about the cooking. It was the entire procedure. I had to come up with two different meals plan for my week. I had to make two separate grocery shopping trips as well as prepare for two meal plans for the week , and cook and clean up for two meals each mealtime! I am a mother of five with five kids and a husband, as well as a cat and a dog. Also, I work. I just did not have the time or energy to keep this amount of work going! I then discovered I could avail AIP meals delivery companies that took care of everything for me! All I needed to do was cook the food they brought to me. It worked for me. There are a variety of delivery services for meals where they provide you with the ingredients that have been prepared along with the recipe, and you cook the food. This can be extremely beneficial for some. Personally, I enjoyed the ability to cook it up and then consume it!

There are a variety of companies to choose from when you choose to go this way. Each one is run slightly differently. You'll have determine what is most effectively for your needs. Are you feeding your entire family using this service or just you? Do you plan to cook or simply cook the food? What is the amount you would like to spend? There are several levels of service, and the prices vary in their prices. Are they able to deliver to my location?

Chapter 7: When Your Self Is Your Own Enemy It Is The Autoimmune Diseases Of Inflammation.

Where did your remarkable immune system originate? "I am awestruck by thee, since I am fearfully and wonderfully made; marvellous work is yours; and my soul is that it is right." The skin of your body is your primary defence. "Every sq inch in your skin comprises of 19 millions cells 60 hairs 90 oil glands 19 inches of blood vessels as well as 625 sweat glands as well as 19,000 sensor cells which can transmit information at speeds of more than 200 miles per hour." Additionally your immune cells on your skin produce antibodies that stop intruders. Not just from the skin, but also from the immune system antibodies are released to protect your sinuses, nasal passages throat, stomach, and intestines. If you did not have these antibodies from your immune system functioning properly and your body, you could be overwhelmed and destroyed. After the skin is covered, the next line of defense lies in your immune system's capacity to launch a full-on defense against all foreign invaders They do, in fact, have a determined and ferocious counter attack. All foreign invaders are able to be identified or not identified. When your body recognizes them (has experienced previously) then it will be able to deal in a more specific and careful manner with the invaders. In the event that your system has not been exposed to them before, it pulls ready with the guns of war and fires everything that is odd. So long as the line of defence removes foreign invaders, you live to be a bit longer and feel content. This defense line is known as inflammation. Inflammation is particularly active to combat any damage, antigen, or virus.

Friendly Fire: What are Autoimmune inflammatory diseases?

If your immune system is compromised, it is unable to effectively fight off diseases and antigens in the normal healthy manner, it must use inflammation to treat the problem. The damage to tissues usually occurs when the body attempts to get rid of invading foreign agents (diseases). However, if the only weapon that can be used is a sledgehammer damage is inevitable. Autoimmune inflammatory disorders can arise in many circumstances in which your immune system isn't functioning at its best. Inflammation can happen when: your immune system isn't functioning at its best and your immune system is misled by foreign antigens from hostile sources or your system's immune response is stimulated too much and the inflammatory process of your immune system is secretly activated and/or your system's immune response is overwhelmed by oxidative stress or other causes of inflammation. There are a few instances of autoimmune diseases that are triggered by the conditions of polymyalgia rheumatica, rheumato and psoriasis, as well as ankylosing spond as well as polyarteritis, scleroderma as well as inflammatory bowel diseases, Crohn's disease, ulcerative colon Irritable bowel, certain instances that are type 1 diabetes chronic fatigue syndrome or multi-sclerosis (MS) as well as systemic lupus erythematosus chronic fatigue and asthma and asthma, among others. If your immune system is weak and can't deal with infection and antigens in the normal healthful way, it turns to chronic inflammation.

What can compromise your immune System? The list of things that could compromise your immune system, causing it reverts to less sophisticated methods of protecting your body's health can be a long list. Here are some of the ones that are the most frequently used and thought as the least hazardous:

The aging immune system As you get older, your immune system is likely to lose its ability to detect autoimmune illnesses more likely. Perhaps you are wondering, "There is nothing I can do to stop my age!" But, as you'll discover, your age can affect you to a greater or lesser extent.

Stressing your body's defenses Stress basically causes the immune system of your body to take a suicide. Stress or burnout from work causes inflammation, which increases your risk of suffering from cardiovascular disease and autoimmune inflammation. If you've experienced significant stress-inducing life events in the last two years, it can increase your chance to develop an auto-immune inflammatory disorder or disorder by 140%!!

Anti-oxidants - A lack of anti-oxidants can cause an increase in oxidative stress. Oxidative stress destroys cells. the immune system produces antibodies to the DNA that has been spilled. The majority of autoimmune inflammation conditions can be diagnosed with the help of DNA antibodies.

Heavy Metal Blues - Heavy metals can cause inflammation in your body which increases the chance of contracting autoimmune inflammatory illnesses. Top heavy metal enemies include mercury, lead beryllium, nickel cobalt, chromium vanadium and cadmium. Mercury increases the severity of your inflammatory tissue damage by up to 50%. (That is the reason why the author had all his mercury fillings taken out!)

A drug-induced Immune System - Many medications are recognized as as risk factors in these autoimmune disorders. For instance, estrogens increase releases of inflammation-related mediators by white cells of the immune system. Contraceptives that are oral increase the risk of developing an autoimmune disease by 90 percent. The hormone replacement therapy can increase the risk of autoimmune inflammatory diseases by 150 percent. The pharmaceutical drugs aren't the only source for these hormones. Animal and chemical products are also significant sources of hormones and similar substances that could cause numerous autoimmune inflammation conditions.

Better "Living" by Chemistry? There are a myriad of harmful chemicals, particularly in work environments that can greatly increase the risk of developing an autoimmune inflammation disorder. For instance, hair products particularly dyes increase the likelihood of having an autoimmune disease by 90 percent. Another reason can be Sodium Lauryl Sulphate (SLS) that lowers the body's defenses to antigen-induced inflammation and also triggers inflammation. SLS is the main commonly used ingredient in toothpaste, shampoos and other personal hygiene products. What do you eat? Food preservatives, such as BHA (3-tert- butyl-4-hydroxyanisole), and food additives, such as emulsifiers, thickeners, surface-finishing agents and contaminants like plasticizers can trigger inflammation in your body. Are you eating crackers along with your soup? The stomach's role is to make acid to aid in digesting your meals. When alkali-containing substances like baking soda/powder is consumed like biscuits, crackers and cakes, your stomach must perform twice as hard to produce the same amount of acidity. Baking powder intake is linked to a 190% rise in the risk of developing stomach cancer. This is usually resulting from an increase in stomach acidity, inflammation and irritation. Toxins and waste materials are removed through the skin. It is recommended to avoid work that causes sweat , and consequently the pores on their skin become blocked with waste. This means that more pressure is put on their bowels, livers and kidneys to eliminate these. This causes increased inflammation as well as increased the risk of liver, skin, and kidney problems. A healthy skin can help fight inflammation-related diseases. Skin hygiene can require thorough scrubbing as well as sweating. Are Your Foods Fresh or is it rotten or out of date? Are you able to find any decent healthy, nutritious food inside a trash can that's dirty? Aflatoxins that are produced during the process of ageing or fermenting can be a significant cause in chronic inflammation. Aflatoxins in the diet include wine, cheese vinegar, wine, and any other food product that has been rotting or fermentation. Researchers use vinegar-based solutions that are weak to induce inflammatory bowel diseases in rodents to study Crohn's disease and ulcerative colitis in humans. Additionally certain chemicals created when foods are picked could increase oxidative stress and inflammation, which can lead to autoimmune diseases and cancer.

Another cause of exposure to aflatoxin can be found in the environmental. Mold and mildew in the air increase the risk of developing autoimmune inflammatory 180% for your lungs, and 360% for joints. Shade trees and trees are close to and thick around houses or building, water damaged structures decaying leaves, sauna baths, compost heaps and wet basements, swamps and lowlands--all are sources for inflammation and aflatoxins. Avoid all mold and decay which are environmental or personal. A healthy lifestyle is dependent on a perfect circulation - Inflammation is more prevalent when blood flow becomes slow and congested. In the end, the risk of developing autoimmune inflammation is more likely to occur with a restless lifestyle, tight clothing , or extremities that are cold. However the moment circulation speeds up and inflammation is reduced, it can be a good thing. In colder weather having short sleeves, or short-length pants can expose your limbs to cooling, which chills the blood returning from the extremities back to the abdomen, chest and pelvis, which is where inflammation may develop. In addition, your clock of the circadian cycle (your inner equilibrium timer that regulates your body's balance of inflammation as well as anti-inflammatory) is disrupted, and inflammatory mediators are released and your risk of developing an autoimmune inflammation rises. Studies have shown that tight clothing can have a negative impact on the body. From slow digestion of food to the increase of the production of inflammatory mediators, wearing tight clothes can increase one's likelihood of suffering from autoimmune inflammatory diseases. Another way that circulation is not in balance and may cause inflammation is due to the overwork in your brain. In fact, over-working your brain without adequate physical activity outdoors always results in an increase in inflammation. Inflammatory illnesses are more frequent in those who perform mental tasks compared to those who perform physical work.

Sleeping off Autoimmune Diseases Sleep loss is linked with the development of autoimmune diseases and increased inflammation. Numerous factors can impact the quality of your sleep and consequently influence your risk of developing autoimmune diseases.

The Air Quality Control - Your indoor air contains more pollutants than outdoor air. Indoor air pollutants are an excellent cause of inflammation. The contaminants include dust that is breathable nitrogen dioxide, chemical compounds such as formaldehydeand Aspergillus aflatoxins as well as various molds.

Avoid letting any illness get out of hand Certain triggers of autoimmune inflammation begin in a small way and gradually grow over time, eventually becoming more than you expected. Poor application of voice or straining your voice poor or ineffective breathing could all lead to inflammation of the throat and lungs which increases the risk of developing the autoimmune inflammation illnesses. Repeated or vigorous tasks can cause tissues micro-traumas, which can cause inflammation which can then be spread throughout your body, increasing your risk of inflammations that are autoimmune.

Spices and Condiments The strong flavor of spice and condiments in the diet can cause inflammation, which can trigger autoimmune diseases. Minice cakes, muffins preserves, meats that are highly-seasoned with pickles, gravies, too much salt and grease as well as mustard, pepper, ketchup and many more. Salt intake that is excessive can cause the risk of renal damage and hypertension due to inflammation and oxidative stress in the blood vessels and kidneys. Black and red peppers dramatically increases the acidity of your stomach, which leads to cell death as well as micro-bleeding and inflammation. Red pepper boosts the amount of stomach acid excreted 700%.

Stimulants Caffeine and its kin could increase the risk of contracting an autoimmune disease. When inflammation begins to develop within your body, caffeine may increase it by 300% to 60 percent. The risk of developing a disease is increased to 150%. while cola drinks increase it by 120%, and coffee by 118 percent. Does alcohol impair your immune system? Drinking alcohol can increase free radicals and causes body inflammation. The effects of wine can be particularly aggravated which can worsen the severity of inflammatory illnesses such like asthma.

Tobacco smoking (even inhaling secondhand smoke) increases inflammation and a depletion of your body's anti-oxidant defenses. It's well-known that smoking cigarettes can have negative effects on many inflammation-related diseases, such as multiple sclerosis, rheumatoid arthritis and inflammatory bowel diseases. Toxic fumes and caustic chemical generated by smoking tobacco increase the chance of contracting immune-mediated inflammatory disorders. The chance of developing an autoimmune inflammation disease increases by at 65% when you smoke and 98% with drinking alcohol. Since the beginning of time, we've known that smoking cigarettes can cause injury and kill people. But, smoking cigarettes is the most common cause of deaths that can be prevented across the U.S. and yet 42.1 million people are smoking and start smoking every day. Are you truly ready to stop? A recent study within the New England Journal of Medicine offers promising results. Examining more than 2,500 participants within the CVS Caremark program, that study showed that those who had an incentive from their personal finances to quit smoking experienced remarkable successes, at minimum after 12 weeks of trying. The most effective program involved smokers deposited 150 of their personal cash first. This person would then receive that $150 plus an additional $650 in the event that they were able to stop smoking. The participants in this program also received advice about quitting, access an online counseling program for free, and were provided with nicotine replacement therapy such as chewing gum or patches. In the end, 52.3% quit. The second largest group of people to quit smoking, received an incentive of $800 (without needing to pay any money of their own) and all the other sources. It was only 17.1 percent of this group succeeded in quitting smoking despite a more potential financial rewards or payouts However, this group also did not risk any losses to their private funds. (Note that the "carrot as well as the whip" is a phrase that roots from earlier "horse and buggy" times of. The cart driver would attach an orange to the end of a stick and hang it before

177

the donkey or horse that is pulling the cart. When the donkey moved toward the carrot it would push the cart as well as the driver since the carrot was always out of reach. If the animal became tired of chasing and pulling a carrot that was unable to be getting further away, a quick hit with the whip could be used to get it moving back. In order to be motivated enough to make progress it is obvious that we need both a whip from behind and the lure of a carrot at to our sides.)

Fast Food And Autoimmune Inflammatory Conditions - Fried potatoes, sweets, salty snacks along with processed foods are some of the most significant causes of increased oxygenation and chronic inflammation. Do you know a single commercial snack which is healthy? Western Diet Woes -A number of studies have found the western diet (described by various names as including: red processed meat, grain-fed meat hot dogs, pork butter, lard hydrogenated fats high saturated fats eggs, high-fat dairy, French fries, potatoes as well as diet and regular soft drinks pizza refined grains, pastas and breads along with tea and coffee sweets/candy, and sweets) and increase the risk of developing autoimmune illnesses by up to 210 percent.

Chapter 8: Restorative And Maintenance Of Your Health Immune System

How do you effectively and safely efficiently restore your weak immune system and keep it in good health condition that will ensure the prevention of any more chronic inflammatory illnesses or their complications, as well as the associated symptoms or pain?

Clean Morning Air Jobs that require physical activity outdoors are extremely protective, whereas living and working in artificial, heated or air-conditioned areas increase the chance of contracting an autoimmune disease. The most efficient immune boosters is a walk in the early morning through the open air close to the body of water, at the time that the sun rises. Have You and Your Body Actually Been To the Sun recently? Exposure to sunlight can decrease inflammation within your body. Because exposure to sunlight is an important source of Vitamin D as well as Vitamin D deficiency can increase the chance of contracting various common inflammatory diseases, e.g. cancers and MS (MS) and rheumatoid arthritis hypertension or cardiovascular heart disease, as well as type I diabetes. It is suggested that at minimum 25 percent of your skin is exposed to sun for at least 20 minutes every day, and more in the case of darker skin.

What is Proper Exercise? Exercise tips the inflammatory/anti-inflammatory balance in favor of reduced inflammation and reduced disease risk. There are a few exceptions to this, however those suffering from autoimmune inflammatory illnesses benefit greatly from regular physical exercise. This leads to significant improvement in strength, pain and fatigue, and does not make their illness worse. As we age, our immune systems diminish. Physical fitness can help slow the decline. Your immune system is responsive to moderate exercise. However, exercising too often can decrease it. When you're working out, loose clothing is more beneficial than clothing that hinders your movements and blood flow. Close fitting clothing has been proven to trigger body temperature fluctuations and interfere with normal circulation of blood and hormonal levels. All of which are components that can be implicated in autoimmune inflammation diseases.

Circadian The Body's Internal Clock. Your organs runs through its internal clock. The anti-inflammatory/inflammatory balance cycles on your clock are called your circadian rhythm. The anti-inflammatory circadian clock is affected when meals are not consistent or meals are eaten late at night or your sleeping hours are inconsistent, inadequate or shift to a later time for bed and/or an early rise time, which is a task that frequently involves shifts where the schedule of your day can change on certain days, like on weekends and days off. Regularity in your sleeping schedule enhances your sleep quality and has an anti-inflammatory effect. For anyone suffering from autoimmune inflammation it is recommended to keep a strict plan for your sleep hours, with an established bedtime for your night that is not later than 9:45 p.m. as well as an established daily rise time of between 7.5 to 8 hours earlier on weekdays and on weekends. Try to maintain regular meals throughout the week that do not vary by more than 5 minutes , and no meal that is that is later than 5:15 p.m. It is important to exercise consistently throughout the week, even on weekend days and days off.

Your diet choices - A research was conducted to compare 4 diet choices: (1) fats and processed meats diet (fats oil prepared meats, fritters potato, desserts and salty snacks) our western diet (2) tomatoes, beans and refined grains (beans tomatoes, beans refined grains, beans, and dairy products with high fat content) an alleged Mediterranean similar diet, (3) seafood and vegetable diet (fish and dark-yellow, dark-cruciferous, and various other vegetables) sea food diet as well as (4) whole fruits and grains (whole grains, fruits nuts, the green leaves of vegetables) Vegan or vegetarian diet. The western diet increased three indicators of inflammation, and the so-called Mediterranean diet increased one indicator of inflammation and the seafood diet reduced one indicator of inflammation, and the vegan or vegetarian diet decreased four indicators of inflammation which shows the immense advantages of a vegan diet when it comes to combating autoimmune diseases.

The Vegetarian Advantage A vegan diet is proven to be anti-inflammatory on people suffering from active autoimmune inflammatory disorders. A vegetarian diet boosts the immune system, boosts the resistance to harmful substances that are found in less healthy diets and is brimming with anti-oxidant anti-inflammatory vitamins as well as phytochemicals. Another benefit of the vegetarian diet is the high levels of natural antioxidants. Research has shown that people with autoimmune diseases consume significantly less anti-oxidant food. But research shows that a high antioxidant intake can significantly reduce your body's inflammation. There's an advantage in eating organic fruit and vegetables. The fruits and vegetables are rich in flavonoids, phytochemicals , and anti-oxidants , which have been proven to decrease your oxidative stress as well as inflammation and the burning of fats (fats) within your body. Also, fruits and vegetables are rich in Vitamin A. Insufficient vitamin A levels leave your body exposed to inflammation caused by oxidative stress as well as autoimmune illnesses. Vitamin A-rich foods comprise sweet potatoes, carrots spinach, kale and winter squash, as well as cantaloupe , and broccoli. Whole grains and fiber can be included in an inflammation-fighting diet. A diet high in whole grains are proven to provide protection against systemic inflammation , which reduces the risk of developing autoimmune diseases. The fiber found in whole grain foods and bran, helps reduce inflammation in people suffering from chronic inflammatory conditions.

What is a low-carb diet to reduce chronic inflammation? High carbohydrate, low fat diets have been found to reduce the body's inflammation. What is the diet that provides the highest amount of anti-oxidant and anti-inflammatory effects? Fresh organic food is the most efficient. Fresh food is a raw vegan diet made up of fruits, berries, root vegetables, as well as nuts sprouts, seeds that have germinated and sprouts, i.e. abundant sources of carotenoids and vitamin C and E (some refer to this as raw-food diet). Fresh food diet have been proven to experience improvements in the symptoms of autoimmune inflammatory diseases like stiff joints as well as sleep quality good health, cholesterol, and weight control. Another factor to consider could be the positive health effects associated with omega-3 acid. Omega-3 fatty acids have been associated with less inflammation, improved in symptoms of illness, and decreased chance of developing autoimmune illnesses. The best sources for omega-3 fats include the vegetarian diet as well as olives, flax, and olive seeds. Olive oil and olives, due to their high concentrations of anti-oxidants, omega-3 fat acids and phytochemicals have been proven to be beneficial in the treatment and prevention of various autoimmune diseases. The most effective method to get the olive oil is through the consumption fresh olives. The results aren't immediate, but generally felt after 12 weeks. A good source of vitamin C is citrus juice and lemon juice. Citrus is rich in phytochemicals, bioflavonoids and anti-oxidants. They have been shown to lower inflammation and ease signs of diseases. Protein consumption can cause negative effects on the potential the autoimmune inflammatory disease sufferer. All proteins are not designed to be the same. Soy Protein (non GMO) reduces your chance of contracting autoimmune inflammatory diseases by 60% when compared with an animal-based diet protein.